PROSTATE PROBLEMS

The complete guide to their treatment

Jeremy Hamand

Thorsons
An Imprint of HarperCollins*Publishers*

Thorsons
An Imprint of GraftonBooks
A Division of HarperCollins*Publishers*
77-85 Fulham Palace Road,
Hammersmith, London W6 8JB

Published by Thorsons 1991
10 9 8 7 6 5 4 3 2 1

A catalogue record for this book
is available from the British Library

ISBN 0 7225 2252 5

Printed in Great Britain by
Woolnough Bookbinding Limited,
Irthlingborough, Northamptonshire

Contents

Foreword

Medicine is now becoming such a rapidly developing and highly technological arena that the journalist is playing an increasingly important role in publicizing new developments, not only to the public but also to the medical profession itself.

Traditionally British patients have been very much more acquiescent and far less well informed than their counterparts in the United States or Continental Europe. Uninformed patients cannot be expected to have a realistic perspective on their treatment, and they are likely to feel the sense of betrayal of trust with their medical advisers. I therefore welcome a trend towards patients becoming increasingly aware of the range of the possible treatments and of the potential problems associated with them.

There can be few problems associated with the human condition which occur as commonly as prostate disorders. Fifty per cent of the population are at risk. Approximately one in five of all males in the United States are liable to have a prostate operation for obstuctive problems during their lifetime, and it has been estimated that half of all elderly males have symptoms which can be ascribed to the prostate.

In addition to obstuctive problems, there are other disorders causing chronic and sometimes disabling pain, which are described by the umbrella term *prostatitis*. Cancer of the prostate also occurs relatively frequently in older men; it varies from a comparatively benign condition to one which has a very much more rapid progression.

Despite the common nature of these complaints, the general knowledge about the prostate in the community is virtually nil, and it is therefore not surprising that advice given to patients in outpatient clinics or doctors' practices is staggeringly unsophisticated. Many patients are likely to be inhibited about asking questions relating to their sexual function, and yet these are vital issues which should be raised at any discussion about prostate surgery.

At last we have a book which gives a clear description of the prostate and what goes wrong with it, and a clear account of the range of treatments which are available for the obstruction caused by benign enlargement, and for prostatitis and cancer.

Prostatic surgery for urinary obstruction has developed enormously over the course of this century, and we urologists now have a treatment which is remarkably effective and which has a very good safety record. However, it is a sledge-hammer which probably isn't required to crack every nut. There are certainly cases where the bladder is so severely obstructed that surgery is unquestionably required. But for the majority of patients it is a very fine line which they cross when they develop sufficiently severe symptoms to warrant surgery. There may be a large number of cases where surgery could be avoided by using alternative treatments. In my opinion, these alternatives are inferior in many respects to prostate surgery, but they are far less gruelling for the patient.

In this book, the reader will find very detailed descriptions of all the alternatives to a full-blown prostatic operation. But he may have to pass on his copy of this book to his doctor, for most of the alternative treatments to prostate surgery are too recent to be included in current medical textbooks. The latest treatments for prostatitis and prostate cancer are also described. I do not know of any other source which covers all these aspects of treatment in one volume.

There are certain misconceptions which are rife among medical practitioners other than urologists. There are many patients who are fobbed off by their doctors because they do not have very enlarged prostates. Conversely, many patients are referred to urologists because their prostates are too large, even though they are causing no symptoms whatsoever. This nonsensical approach reflects the sad level of training and the perpetuation of totally outmoded concepts. This book addresses many such misconceptions.

I therefore strongly recommend that it be widely read. While many doctors will certainly gain some useful insight from several of these chapters, actual and potential sufferers from prostatic disorders will be forearmed and will approach any treatment with far more understanding, and therefore with far less anxiety.

Finally, the reader will learn from these pages that there are many new treatments on the horizon, and many of these will find an established place for treating prostatic problems, including prostatitis and possibly cancer. My prediction is that routine prostatic surgery for urinary obstuction will still be with us in one or two decades' time, but that it will be used for only the most refractory cases. The urologist will be relying primarily on tablets and a variety of high-technology manipulations for treating 90 per cent of prostate sufferers.

Graham Watson MD, FRCS
Consultant and Senior Lecturer, Institute of Urology

Introduction

Most men reach middle age with only a vague idea of what or even where the prostate gland is. They will have heard it mentioned – often in terms of awe and apprehension – by relatives discussing old Uncle So-and-so's problems or Grandpa's operation. They may have a vague knowledge of the prostate's connections with ejaculation and fertility.

But by the time a man reaches his mid-50s or early-60s, the word 'prostate' starts to take on a more real meaning for him: one or two of his contemporaries are reported to 'have prostate problems' or even to have 'had their prostate out'. It begins to dawn on him that his prostate, too, is a potential source of problems, and he becomes fearful of medical examinations in case he too is found to have an enlarged prostate, and may worry that his urination is showing signs of abnormality.

What goes wrong with the prostate? What are the symptoms? What treatment is available? What happens when the prostate is 'removed'? Most importantly, for most men, how is one's sex life likely to be affected?

The answers to these and similar questions are not that easy to come by. Sometimes a good GP, if he has time, can explain things. But little written information is available for the general reader. There are no 'Well Man' clinics where such things can be talked over. Newspapers and magazines, put off perhaps by a subject combining excretion and sexual function, fight shy of features or advice columns on prostate problems, although few dispense with lengthy articles on various aspects of women's health and reproductive problems. For similar reasons, friends may not be keen to discuss the issue, and are in any case unlikely to be well-informed.

Hence the justification for this book, which aims to give information and explanations, but not to be a self-treatment guide. Fear of doctors and hospitals is often fuelled by ignorance of what has gone wrong with one's bodily functions and uncertainty about how medical treatment can help put things to rights.

Successive chapters of this book will describe the function of the prostate (as far as it is understood by medical science), the three main diseases of the gland, and the range of conventional treatments currently available. It will also outline some of the 'alternative' treatments which have been developed, and look at some of the more promising experimental treatments being tried out.

What most people understand by prostate trouble is caused by the common condition of 'benign enlargement'. This enlargement, or hyperplasia, which occurs in almost all men in middle or old age, sometimes makes the prostate press on the urethra and on the bladder sphincter, reducing the flow of urine. This process does not of itself interfere with sexual activity, since the gland continues to function much as before. But if the obstruction progresses beyond a certain point, the bladder ceases to empty properly. This in turn causes certain symptoms, and if untreated, can lead to serious bladder problems, the formation of bladder stones, and kidney damage caused by back pressure from the bladder.

The conventional medical treatment is to remove the obstructing tissue (not the complete prostate gland), which normally reduces or eliminates symptoms and, more importantly, prevents damage (or further damage) to the bladder and kidneys. The operation does not directly affect sexuality, but a common side-effect is the ejaculation of semen backwards into the bladder at orgasm, instead of out through the penis in the usual way.

'Prostatitis' is a catch-all term used to describe infection, inflammation or pain in the prostate, which can arise from a number of different causes and, at one time or another in their lives, affects large numbers of men, often when they are still young. Some types of prostatitis clear up quickly and easily, but others are extremely difficult to treat, and can continue to torment their sufferers for years or decades. An operation is not usually the answer.

Cancer (or carcinoma) of the prostate is very common in elderly men, but often creates no symptoms or problems. But some forms of the cancer do create urinary obstruction, and therefore urologists always try to rule out cancer before diagnosing benign enlargement. Treatment and prognosis, as with most cancers, depend on the extent of the disease when it is diagnosed: among them are radiotherapy by external beam or by radioactive needles implanted in the prostate, hormones (since prostate cancer growth is dependent on male hormones) and complete removal of the prostate gland. Sometimes, the cancer progresses only very slowly, and in such cases it may be felt best not to try to treat it at all, but just monitor its progress.

All three diseases described above are relatively common. According to the US National Institutes of Health, 'more than 80 per cent of adult males 50–60 years of age have benign enlargement of the prostate gland' – the proportion rising with age – and at least 10 per cent of them will require surgery. Every year some 50,000 men in Britain and 300,000 in the United States have a prostate operation, mainly for benign enlargement; and for every man operated on, another half dozen will see their doctors with prostate symptoms requiring treatment or monitoring.

In fact, the problem is even bigger than that, since many men put off seeing their doctors, and urologists estimate that as many as half a million men in Britain may be suffering from prostate symptoms at any one time. In the United States, with its much larger population, there are probably around 3 million such men.

Prostate surgery is the most commonly performed urological operation, yet on average National Health Service patients in Britain will wait five to eight months for a non-urgent prostate operation, which may be extended in some areas to as long as five years. Some British hospitals have simply stopped doing non-urgent prostate operations at all. Not a few British men die of other causes while on hospital waiting lists – one explanation of why the proportion of men receiving prostate surgery in Britain is much lower than in the United States.

The drain on health service resources is enormous. In Britain about 76 beds per million adult men are needed for diseases of the prostate (mainly benign enlargement) at any one time; and about 90 of every 10,000 men over the age of 65 are admitted for these diseases every year. The annual overall cost of hospital care and surgery for benign enlargement alone in the United States is over a billion dollars.

Prostatitis is described as one of the commonest reasons for men to visit their doctor. And prostate cancer is the second most frequent fatal cancer among men in North America. In the developing countries, where prostate diseases have remained largely untreated up till now, the 2,000 million males now alive will live longer than their fathers and grandfathers, and benign enlargement and prostate cancer will become much more frequent because their incidence rises sharply with age. So the need for cheaper, less invasive treatment is going to rise in parallel with the increase in the numbers of elderly men.

Existing treatment is imperfect – although a great advance on only 20 or 30 years ago. Unfortunately, many myths persist about the prostate and treatment for its diseases. And for some reason men are less likely than women are to discuss their health problems with friends or relatives.

So it is scarcely surprising that men don't like to talk about their prostate problems (touching as they do on sex and excretion), and – notoriously – put off seeing their doctors when they develop urinary difficulties. This sometimes means that they have to be treated for acute symptoms – even given emergency surgery – which is inevitably more traumatic than learning to understand a chronic complaint and being kept under observation.

In recent years, prominent politicians such as President Ronald Reagan, Chancellor Helmut Kohl and Australian Prime Minister Bob Hawke have had their prostate problems – successfully treated – exposed to the glare of publicity. But in one famous case, a politician's failure to consult his doctor in time probably resulted in the premature end to his career and may even have altered history. This was the British Prime Minister Harold Macmillan, who when struck down by acute symptoms and faced with an immediate operation, became convinced he was dying of cancer, and decided to resign, cursing 'this filthy disease'. He never developed cancer, and lived for another 25 years, regretting his precipitate decision (see Chapter 1).

There is another reason apart from prudishness why men put off seeing their doctors for symptoms which have developed gradually and may not be too difficult to ignore. This is that they suspect, and on the whole they are correct, that they are likely to have to have a major operation which can have unpleasant side-effects.

It is true that the only conventional treatment for severe urinary obstruction caused by an enlarged prostate gland is the surgical removal of most of the gland. While as we shall see in Chapter 3, the operation is far less serious, far safer and has fewer side-effects than was the case 50 years ago, it remains a major operation, and although the dreaded side-effects of impotence and incontinence are now mercifully very rare, the operation remains a threat to fertility. This is not because it prevents a man producing sperm, but because it often happens that (as described above) after the operation semen is ejaculated backwards into the bladder ('retrograde ejaculation').

This is of more concern today than in the past because the improved safety of the operation has meant that more younger men are given the operation to prevent them developing acute symptoms. Another factor is the higher divorce rate, which has resulted in more older men marrying second wives who are still in the fertile age range and may well want to have children.

Bearing in mind the huge numbers of men receiving the operation nowadays – numbers that are likely to increase exponentially in the coming decades as men live longer in the developing countries – it is hardly surprising that there is a flourishing prostate 'industry', with many conferences taking place and books and papers published in attempts to refine treatment. The development of an effective non-surgical treatment would of course be an amazing leap forward – promising a fortune to the company which develops the successful pill or device – and we will be looking at some of the attempts to improve surgery and develop outpatient treatments later in this book.

Alternative medicine, such as homoeopathy and naturopathy, offers non-surgical treatments, but in Britain the medical establishment tends to be wary of these, if not positively disparaging, pointing out that prostate conditions sometimes improve spontaneously, for a while at least, or when treated with placebo pills. But other countries look more sympathetically on them, and in France and West Germany, for instance, there are several herbal remedies which are actually prescribed by conventional urologists (see Chapter 7).

Some may really help, in so far mainly unexplained ways, to stem the development of prostatic disease, although no alternative treatment could claim to be a cure: such a development would be front-page news! But there has been little scientific assessment of such treatments, and the prostate sufferer should not expect too much of them. For some people, however, faced with a long wait for a prostate operation, such remedies may be attractive and may help provide some relief in the meantime, as well as making a man feel he is at least doing something to help his condition.

One difficulty for both the urologist and his patient is to know when it is best to operate. While some cases are clear-cut, in that the severe kidney damage or even death will shortly follow if surgery is not performed, most cases are more complex. The decision to operate or not must be taken by the surgeon on the basis of his assessment of likely damage to the bladder or kidneys if the condition continues uncorrected, and also on the basis of the patient's perception of his symptoms and how much they interfere with his lifestyle.

It is usually impossible to predict whether or how quickly a patient's symptoms are likely to deteriorate. Sometimes a man with moderately severe symptoms will not get much worse over a long period, while a man with less severe symptoms suddenly finds himself in need of emergency treatment. The surgeon may also not be sure how much improvement the operation will bring, especially if the patient complains of severe symptoms while his condition appears to the surgeon not to be too serious.

Urologists themselves, being only human, may vary considerably in their assessment of the same case. Some are known to be of the 'Let's get cracking' school, believing that the risks of the operation are almost always less than the risks of kidney damage. Others are often reluctant to operate unless absolutely necessary, and prefer to keep patients under observation, perhaps for years. Every operation has its risks, and a urologist may feel it's not worth taking that risk and hope the man's condition does not get too much worse.

While your urologist's particular approach may be an unknown factor, it certainly always helps to understand something of the anatomy of prostate complaints, to know what options the urologist may have in mind, and to be familiar with some of the medical terminology likely to be used. Then you have a better chance of asking the right questions and of understanding the answers.

Frank B. of London, who had a prostate operation when he was 66, was puzzled when told by the consultant afterwards that 'Nothing was found.' What could be meant? No prostate? No stones? No diamonds?! Mr B. was not to know (since he was not told) that prostate tissue removed in an operation is always checked for latent cancer cells, and the surgeon was simply reassuring him that no cancer was present. The urologist's routine check and routine reassurance had no meaning for him.

'The more I think on this topic,' writes Mr B., 'the more I realize how little information was volunteered. I am sure that I would have received answers if I had asked questions. Fortunately I appear to be in reasonably good health, rather old-fashioned and therefore not versed in bodily functions – unlike many of my younger friends.'

But Mr B. is perhaps overestimating the knowledge of his younger friends. How many would know exactly where the prostate is and how it causes problems? Or have heard of, never mind understand, 'retrograde ejaculation' (explained above), 'nocturia' (getting up in the night to pee), 'indwelling catheter' (permanently fitted tube to drain the bladder), 'urethral stricture' (narrowing of the urethra), 'residual volume' (amount of urine left in the bladder after urinating), 'cystoscopy' (visual examination of the inside of the bladder) and the other medical jargon that doctors use amongst themselves and in their notes, if not to their patients?

American doctors are mainly better at explaining things, perhaps because their patients are paying them fees directly. But British patients should not forget that they have a right to medical information from their doctors' files.

Mr B.'s experience – of how little information was volunteered – will strike a chord in all too many patients who have seen consultants, whether for prostate or other health problems.

This is unfortunate, since recent studies have shown that men are least likely to have sexual problems after prostate surgery if the nature of the operation and its effects are fully explained to them, while men who undergo surgery in ignorance have more problems afterwards than is usual. The message of such research will not be lost on urologists, but the profession is a conservative one and changes in attitude are slow to take effect.

A man with a general grasp of what has gone wrong with his body, what his symptoms mean, and what can be done to help him, will face his consultant with more confidence and better equipped to ask questions. As long as his approach is not aggressive or 'know-all', the specialist is likely to treat him with greater respect, and perhaps even show relief to find a patient who has an informed interest in his condition.

So a final aim of this book is to provide the prostate sufferer with the background and information to talk sensibly and confidently to his doctor and consultant.

CHAPTER 1

What does the prostate do, and what goes wrong?

The prostate is a curious piece of anatomy. Most mammals have one in some form, yet its function is little understood. In the words of one expert, 'it is not essential for life and is associated in some way with reproduction, but even for this it is not essential.' Like that of the appendix, the role of the prostate remains obscure.

The male reproductive and urinary systems

It will help you to understand what follows if you have a basic understanding of the structure and function of the male reproductive organs and the kidneys, bladder and urinary system and see how they all fit together.

The prostate gland is situated just below the bladder, fitting like a collar round the urethra, the tube which carries urine from the bladder down through the penis to the outside. The Greek words from which 'prostate' was derived by the 16th-century French surgeon Ambroise Paré imply the function of 'door-keeper' to the bladder. Urinating is controlled by two sphincter muscles, an external one which is under voluntary control, and an internal one which closes to prevent sperm being ejaculated backwards into the bladder when a man ejaculates – or urine being mixed with the semen. Two ureters, one from each kidney, join the bladder, and it is along these that the urine passes before being stored in the bladder.

The kidneys are responsible for filtering various waste products out of the blood; the result is urine, which contains urea and other compounds which would be toxic if they remained in the body. The kidneys can only work effectively if the pressure outside them is lower than inside; if urine is allowed to build up in the ureters because the bladder cannot be emptied properly, the kidneys can no longer filter out the harmful substances efficiently. This can result in uraemic poisoning, which causes the patient to become ill and weak and finally results in death.

The urethra, leading from the bladder to the outside through the penis, also carries the semen and sperm during ejaculation. Sperm are produced in the testes in long convoluted tubes called the seminiferous tubules. They are then stored in the epididymis. They can also be temporarily stored at the top of the vasa deferentia, the tubes which lead from the testes through to the ejaculatory ducts which empty into the urethra inside the prostate gland. When a man is sexually excited, more sperm are pumped up through the vasa deferentia, and during orgasm, sperm, fluid from the seminal vesicles situated at the base of the bladder, and the prostate secretions all pour into the urethra because of contractions of the seminal vesicles and prostate muscles. Muscles surrounding the urethra then contract to expel the semen from the penis at ejaculation.

The prostate is actually not a single gland but a whole bundle of tiny glands arranged in three lobes which discharge their secretions into the urethra on ejaculation. These secretions only make up a small proportion (around 10 per cent) of the total volume of semen ejaculated. The rest of the semen, consisting mainly of the output of the seminal vesicles lying on each side of the bladder, and the sperm itself, pumped up through the vasa deferentia, actually passes in two ducts through the prostate, discharging into the urethra alongside the prostatic ducts.

Prostatic fluid is thought to stimulate or possibly nourish the sperm in some way, but sperm can apparently manage quite well without it. So although the gland may have a marginal effect on male fertility, it is certainly not indispensable.

Prostatic fluid contains a cocktail of enzymes, some substances that neutralize bacteria, citric acid, fructose, zinc, and a group of fluids called (after the gland itself) prostaglandins. These last are hormones which have remarkable pharmacological effects on smooth muscle and blood vessel walls, and are medically used to bring on dilation of the cervix and uterine contractions in childbirth. Prostaglandins are also used to induce labour and to induce abortion.

A recent development of this property has been the perfection of a system to help the 15 per cent of women who experience difficulties in childbirth due to an 'unripened' (insufficiently dilated) cervix. The scientists have developed a capsule of hydrogel polymer containing prostaglandin hormone which is implanted in a woman going into labour, releasing the hormone at a constant rate over several hours. It is hoped that this will usually cut labour by about two-thirds, and reduce the number of women requiring a caesarean. Prostaglandins used in such applications are synthetically manufactured.

One theory about the function of prostatic fluid is that the prostaglandins in it serve to encourage the cervix to dilate very slightly to make it easier for the sperm to pass through the cervix (neck of the womb) into the uterus. The prostatic fluid is in fact usually ejaculated in the first contraction of orgasm, just before the bulk of the semen from the seminal vesicles, so this theory would seem to make sense.

However, whatever its function, the human prostate gland unfortunately is the site of two common diseases – 'benign enlargement' and prostate cancer – which for all practical purposes do not occur in animals. The human prostate is curious in that while it almost always enlarges in middle or old age, it by no means always causes medical problems as it does so; and although it frequently turns malignant in elderly men, it relatively seldom spreads or causes problems, so that as many as three-quarters of men over 70 may have cancer cells in their prostates yet go to their graves without suffering from it or knowing about it. In younger men, it can become infected or inflamed (prostatitis) in a way that is sometimes difficult or impossible to cure.

Although the prostate causes men so much trouble, it poses particular problems for scientists because it is not easily accessible. Other research problems arise because it is made up of a wide variety of cell types, and because animal prostates are different from human prostates. Mammalian prostates differ greatly, and some animals have two or three prostates. Only in a few animals – rats, mice, dogs, guinea-pigs – can anything like human 'benign enlargement' or prostate cancer be induced.

The prostate is also a very variable organ, which enlarges to a different degree in men of the same age, and causes urinary problems to a different degree for the same degree of enlargement.

When the prostate causes trouble, it is not the gland's function on sexual reproduction which goes wrong; it is the effect of the enlarged or ageing gland on the exit from the bladder which causes problems. Some men assume that the prostate is in some way connected with the production of urine, since its enlargement 'makes them go more often'. But there is no direct connection between prostate and kidneys. See Fig. 1.1 for the location of the prostate gland.

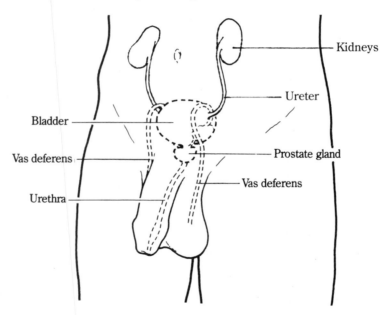

Fig. 1.1: location of prostate gland

When the prostate enlarges, either for benign or malignant reasons, it presses on the urethra and on the bladder neck muscle, and restricts the flow of urine. If the resistance becomes greater than the pressure the bladder muscle is able to exert, then the bladder ceases to empty completely, leaving 'residual urine'. This in turn may build up, and the stagnant urine may become a breeding ground for bacteria which are always present in insignificant numbers in the body, just awaiting a suitable opportunity to multiply. The presence of an infection makes the urine more alkaline, which may encourage calcium salts in the urine to crystallize on an impurity, resulting in a bladder stone, which will increase in size until it causes symptoms of its own.

Most dangerous of all, the obstruction may cause urine to be forced back up the ureters (the tubes that bring the urine from the kidneys), causing back pressure on the kidneys and sometimes infection. The kidneys may then cease to perform their task of purifying the blood properly. This is always the main concern of a urologist facing a patient with urinary problems.

Often, an additional problem is caused by the central or median lobe of the prostate bulging into the bladder, so that the bladder is not able to extend as freely as before, and feels fuller than it really is.

The enlargement and obstruction may build up gradually – over 5, 10 even 20 years – so that the man may sometimes be unaware that he has a potential problem. He may believe that the reduction in his stream is simply something that happens as one gets older. In fact, it does happen that the bladder muscle weakens in older men – but this effect alone is not enough to cause urological problems in the absence of any obstruction. He may well not notice that he is failing to empty his bladder completely when he has a pee; he may forget the feeling of relief and satisfaction which total emptying brings; he may feel no pain or discomfort until, out of the blue, he is stricken with a bladder infection or even acute retention, when he is unable to pass any water at all, even if desperate to do so.

The symptoms of urinary obstruction are unpredictable and sometimes alarming. It helps to have some understanding of why they occur and of the damage to the bladder which results when it is constantly under stress.

Bladder function and malfunction

The bladder consists of a powerful muscle (known as the *detrusor*), two entry valves for the ureters from each kidney, and an exit valve (*internal sphincter*) to the urethra. When urination commences, reflexes cause the bladder sphincter and the external sphincter to relax and the detrusor to contract, forcing the urine out.

Men differ from women in being equipped with two urethral sphincters: the main, 'external' sphincter, just downstream of the prostate, and the bladder sphincter, where the prostate joins the bladder. The function of this extra sphincter is to close off the bladder at orgasm so that the semen is ejaculated outwards through the penis. It is this sphincter which often enlarges with an enlarged prostate, becoming more difficult to open or constricting the urine flow. It is usually removed with the enlarged prostate tissue during a prostatectomy, inevitably causing retrograde ejaculation back into the bladder, the external sphincter shutting off to prevent leakage of urine.

A normal bladder, unobstructed, will expel all the urine in it, and then remain collapsed, more or less flat like an empty football, until refilled from the kidneys. In the case of resistance, whether caused by prostate enlargement or narrowing of the urethra (*stricture*), the bladder at first increases the pressure of its contractions, so that often there is little or no reduction in the stream and no urine left behind.

But as the resistance caused by the growing obstruction increases, the bladder can no longer 'compensate' for the obstruction, and a weaker stream results. Sometimes voiding then becomes incomplete, and *residual urine* or *chronic retention* results.

The slowing of the urine flow rate may happen so slowly that the man never notices it. Usually he does notice it, but is ready to attribute it to 'growing older'. Indeed, the power of the bladder muscle does diminish with age, but this is not sufficient to cause urological problems on its own.

Reduction in the calibre and force of the urine stream are one of the three *primary* symptoms of urinary outflow obstruction. The other two are *delay or hesitancy*, and *terminal dribbling*.

Hesitancy

Hesitancy is an abnormal delay between the release of central inhibition and the start of the stream. Delay may of course be longer in a public place, and some individuals are often 'anxious voiders'. The normal time lapse is only a few seconds, but hesitancy may vary from 10 seconds to several minutes. When the stream does begin, it may ebb and flow, and stop and start, as the bladder muscle tries to contract again and again to empty the remaining urine.

Hesitancy may be caused partly by the time needed to attain the extra pressure within the bladder when there is an outflow obstruction. But this is unlikely to exceed about 10 seconds. In the case of longer hesitancy, it may be that the bladder sphincter takes longer to relax, or that the speed of bladder muscle contraction is slowed. When residual urine remains, the bladder never fully contracts, and so may never fully recover its full expulsive strength.

Terminal dribbling

In a man without an obstruction, the urine flow ends fairly abruptly. But where there is obstruction, the flow may continue at a low level for some seconds. This is because bladder pressure falls towards the end of urination, bringing it into critical balance with the outflow resistance, and, instead of a continuous flow ending abruptly, terminal dribbling occurs. Sometimes the bladder tries to contract once more after the man has 'finished' and returned his penis to his trousers, resulting in damp underwear. This phenomenon tends to be followed by the development of residual urine.

The above are the only *primary* symptoms of urinary obstruction. The *secondary* symptoms are more numerous and on the whole more alarming and more likely to give concern to the patient.

The most common is *frequency*. Frequency of urination depends on fluid intake and its timing, degree of perspiration, ambient temperature (the kidneys are more active in cold weather), amount of exercise taken, and the presence of any infection or a medical condition such as diabetes. Under normal circumstances, the kidneys excrete urine during the day at about 60 ml per hour; the normal bladder begins to signal fullness at over 150 ml, and usual daytime voiding frequency is less than six times a day – an average of about once every three hours.

Men with prostate obstruction often have to go more frequently than this, because if there is residual urine present after urination, the bladder reaches its capacity more quickly; and because an obstructed bladder develops instability and irritability, leading it to signal fullness at smaller volumes.

Another common symptom is getting up in the night (*nocturia*, to a doctor). Normally, the kidneys will produce less urine when a person is asleep, and the bladder will signal 'full' at a larger volume, enabling people to sleep through the night uninterrupted. However, if the bladder is irritable, and/or there is residual urine, the man will be woken by a full bladder sensation.

However, 'getting up' once is not necessarily abnormal, since anyone who drinks a lot in the evening or has a lot of coffee should expect to get up once in the night. Also, older people excrete more urine at night than younger people; and postural changes may also be responsible: fluid that pools in the periphery during the day is redistributed at night and then excreted. But many people with prostatic obstruction have to get up twice or more – and sometimes get no more than two hours' sleep at a stretch, which is very tiring.

Another classical symptom of obstruction is *urgency*, usually caused by the increased irritability of a bladder under stress. An urgent desire to void may come on fairly suddenly, and be so strong that it is sometimes accompanied by a sensation of impending leakage. This symptom can create considerable stress, for the man knows that throughout the day he must be able to have ready access to a lavatory every hour or so. Occasionally, urgency is accompanied by *incontinence* (see Case history 1.1). These symptoms are sometimes caused, and always made worse, by infections of the bladder and urethra, which are common when volumes of urine are habitually retained after voiding. Often, the sound of running water or the sight of a lavatory are enough to set off an 'urgent' signal in an unstable bladder.

An even more distressing symptom is *enuresis* (bed-wetting). This is caused by 'overflow incontinence' which may occur when large volumes of urine are retained and the bladder's 'full' signalling mechanism is disrupted by permanent stretching.

Many men with obstruction experience a *feeling of incomplete emptying* which may or may not reflect the true presence of residual urine. Like most of these symptoms, this feeling is caused not by the pressure of the prostate itself, as is sometimes thought, but simply by an 'irritable' or 'unstable' bladder.

Sometimes there is *pain* on urination, which may or may not be the result of infection. Occasionally some *blood* is passed (*haematuria*). This may be caused by surface veins of the prostate bleeding, but other possible causes need to be investigated, because it may be caused by infection or cancer. So any blood in the urine must always be followed by a visit to the doctor. If blood is passed at the end of urination, accompanied by pain, it is known as *strangury* and is usually a symptom of an infection or *calculus* (stone).

Acute retention is the inability to pass water at all. It is an alarming and dangerous condition that requires prompt medical intervention. It is caused either by an infection developing in retained stale urine which inflames the bladder neck and prostate, blocking the urethra; or by an obstructed bladder being overfilled, with the result that the bladder muscle is stretched so thin that it is weakened and cannot contract enough to force the urine out. This effect can sometimes be noticed when the bladder is full, for example first thing in the morning: the stream is slow to start with, and may even fail to empty the bladder completely.

Drinking alcohol can sometimes trigger an attack of acute retention. This is because alcohol, a central nervous system depressant, both damps down 'full' signals from the bladder so that they go unnoticed, and relaxes and reduces the tone of all muscles – including the bladder. It is also diuretic (tending to make the body excrete more urine), so may encourage the bladder to fill up quickly. Some drugs, such as ephedrine and pseudephedrine, may have similar effects by increasing bladder sphincter resistance, and some anaesthetics and tranquillizing agents may work in the same way, causing acute retention after operations.

If symptoms of obstruction are long ignored, infections of the whole urinary tract and kidneys can result, with fever, aches and pains. Even more seriously, kidney function may be affected, because the kidneys rely on the pressure 'downstream' being lower than the pressure of the blood entering them. Back-pressure up the ureters (ducts from the kidneys to the bladder) then leads to unexcreted waste products being returned to the bloodstream, causing a general feeling of malaise. Chronic renal failure may intervene, causing nausea, vomiting, anorexia (loss of appetite), weight loss, anaemia, apathy and eventually coma.

When the bladder is kept constantly under pressure by a large volume of residual urine, it first thickens in an attempt to expel the urine. This may lead to the formation of small pouches, or saccules, in the spaces between the overlapping bands of muscle fibre – a process known as *trabeculation*. Sometimes these pouches are 'blown out' through the bladder wall to form *diverticula*, rather as blow-outs can form on a tyre. These sacs and pouches are often a focus for infection, and are the most likely place for stones or *calculi* to form, which can lead to further irritation and outflow obstruction. Bladder stones are usually quite small and are easily crushed by an instrument inserted through the urethra, but they can reach a size of an orange, in which case they have to be removed by open surgery.

If symptoms have not been allowed to become too severe or continue over too long a time, many bladder problems (such as irritation and small diverticula) will disappear after a prostatectomy. In many cases, bladder 'instability' proves to be reversible once the obstruction is removed, and so frequency, nocturia and urgency can be expected largely to disappear. But although some men experience rapid relief of their symptoms – perhaps within days of their operation – others may have to wait 12 months or more before very much improvement is noticed. In cases of prolonged retention, when the bladder may have lost its elasticity and be 'like a paper bag' to quote one London urologist, little improvement may ever be seen, and even flow rates will remain sluggish, although normally little urine is retained.

A final word of warning to all who have bladder outflow obstruction: never try to 'improve' your frequency by cutting down on fluid intake. Obviously the amount of urine produced does depend on the quantity of fluid drunk, as well as (among other things) the amount of fluid lost through perspiration. But it certainly does not help by trying to extend the time between 'pees' by drinking less. On the contrary, people with outflow obstruction should drink more, even at the expense of 'going' more often. This is because, where there is residual urine, it is less likely to become infected if it is regularly diluted with fresh urine.

Do not be tempted to hold out as long as possible before

emptying your bladder; and always give yourself as much time as possible to do so: an unhurried bladder will perform more efficiently, so wait until you are sure as you can be that your bladder has finished performing, and identify and wait for the sensation of relief that comes only when the bladder is fully empty. Many men find that they empty their bladders more efficiently when sitting or squatting.

Any extra drinks should not be alcoholic. For the reasons mentioned above, alcoholic intake should be limited if the bladder muscle is not to be weakened, creating a risk of acute retention. And many people find it wise to avoid coffee as well, because coffee often has an irritating effect on the bladder, an effect likely to be more marked if the bladder is already 'unstable'.

When you see your doctor

Confronted with any symptoms short of extreme urgency or acute retention (not being able to pass water at all), many general practitioners will tell the patient to relax and come back if things get worse. They may do a rectal examination, which involves putting a lubricated, rubber-gloved finger up the rectum for a moment to assess the size of the prostate, and also feel the surface of the gland through the bowel wall to see if it is smooth or if there are any corrugations, which might be a sign of malignancy.

If the doctor suspects that the patient has 'chronic retention' (i.e. is regularly not emptying his bladder completely), or has an infection of the urinary tract, or if the patient simply feels his symptoms are intolerable, he will refer him to a urologist. Urologists are consultant surgeons who specialize in diseases of the kidneys, bladder, prostate, urethra, testicles and other parts of the genito-urinary tract. Confronted with a patient who is apparently suffering from urinary obstruction, the urologist will know, if the man is middle-aged or older, that he is probably suffering from an enlarged prostate. But although this is the most likely cause, he must rule out other causes, as well as determining as best he can the degree of obstruction. The tests he is most likely to do are given below (of course, it is unlikely that he will want to do all of them, and may only do one or two).

Rectal digital examination

Examination with one or two forefingers to assess surface texture and size of prostate. Some men dislike this form of penetration, but it doesn't last long, and, as their wives will surely confirm, it is nowhere near as uncomfortable as a female internal examination.

Uroflowmetry

This test is done to establish the speed or calibre of the urine flow ('peak flow rate') and the volume voided. This is simple and painless. It involves urinating (with a full bladder) into either a plastic bottle with a special bypass in it which measures the maximum speed of the flow as well as the total volume; or into the funnel of an electronic device which prints out a graph of the flow pattern, as well as recording the maximum

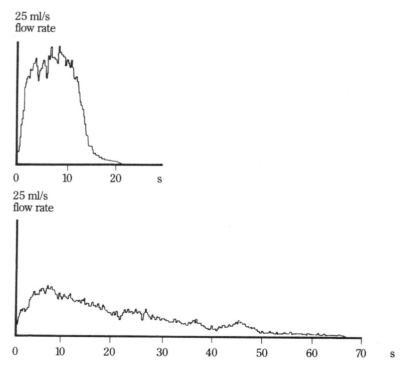

Fig. 1.2: normal flow rate and flow rate with prostate problem

flow rate, time to peak flow, total volume and total time. Peak flow rates depend to a certain extent on age, but generally, a peak flow rate of under 15 ml per second indicates a degree of obstruction. Nobody should consider himself properly evaluated or should agree to prostate surgery without a proper flow rate test being performed.

Urine test

A mid-stream urine sample is analysed to see if it contains blood (haematuria), sugar (diabetes), or is infected.

Blood test

Blood levels of two body waste products, urea and creatinine, are analysed. These products are usually disposed of by the kidneys, and abnormal levels in the blood mean that the kidneys are not functioning properly.

Abdominal examination

The consultant (or GP) may feel the patient's abdomen to check whether his bladder is 'palpable' to the touch. Although a bladder may be difficult to feel unless it is very full, it may make a dull sound when tapped.

Ultrasound examination

The development of ultrasound technology in recent years has proved a real boon to the urologist. Using much the same equipment as is used to check on the development of a foetus in a pregnant woman, an ultrasound technician can now accurately measure how much urine is left in the bladder after urination ('residual urine'), as well as check on the state of the kidneys, ureters and bladder, and the size of the prostate.

Until quite recently, the only way of measuring residual volume was to insert a catheter and drain the bladder into a jug; as well as being rather uncomfortable for the patient, this was always liable to set up an infection, making his condition even worse.

Ultrasound consists of high-frequency sound waves which are bounced off tissues in the body to produce a photographic image on a screen. Unlike X-rays, which have much higher powers of penetration, ultrasound will show up soft tissues and not just bones.

The abdominal ultrasound examination is simple, non-invasive and painless. The technician first scans the patient's stomach with a full bladder by rubbing on a jelly to enable the scanner to make close contact with the skin, then moving a small hand-held device over it. Then the patient empties his bladder and returns for the second scan. The technician calculates the volumes, comments on any abnormalities in the appearance of the bladder or prostate, and provides photostat copies of particular images of significance. The modern ultrasound scan can also show most of the things that the more invasive, more time-consuming and more expensive IVP (see below) used to be used for.

Transrectal ultrasound

This is a more specialized examination, which is sometimes done either to measure the exact dimensions of the prostate, or to check for the presence of prostate stones or small cancerous tumours.

The procedure is rather like the doctor's digital examination. A lubricated finger-shaped metal probe is inserted in the rectum and kept there for a few minutes while the measurements and images are recorded.

Cystoscopy

This is a visual examination of the inside of the urethra and bladder. It is carried out to check for any strictures (see page 73) in the urethra, see the degree to which the prostate is constricting the urethra, and to examine the bladder for any infection or abnormality.

Because it is an invasive procedure and can be unpleasant, it is usually carried out immediately before a prostate operation, while the patient is anaesthetized, but it can be done separately and sometimes afterwards as well. It is not usually performed as an outpatient procedure when there is residual urine in the bladder because of the risk of introducing an infection.

The urologist first squeezes some anaesthetic gel into the

urethra through the penis, then inserts a pencil-thick instrument which is either rigid, or more usually nowadays, flexible and making use of fibre optics, which enable a light source to travel round curves. It is disconcerting and uncomfortable but not really painful, unless there is an infection present. Urologists treat the procedure as routine and certainly nothing to make a fuss about, a view often not shared by their patients, who are often alarmed at the prospect of having a metal tube inserted up their penis when they are anyway likely to be anxious about the operation they are probably facing.

Intravenous pyelogram (IVP)

Sometimes referred to as an 'excretory urogram', this procedure produces an X-ray of the kidneys, ureters and bladder, showing any abnormalities or malignancies. Until recently, it was frequently used to assess the amount of residual urine left after excretion and to check if there was any obstruction to the drainage of the kidneys. Today, these assessments are almost all provided much more cheaply, quickly and pleasantly for the patient by the abdominal ultrasound scan (see above).

This is fortunate, because the IVP is a time-consuming, unpleasant and sometimes dangerous technique which involves the injection into a vein in the forearm of a radioactive isotope of iodine which concentrates in the kidneys. After a wait to allow the kidneys to collect enough dye, a series of X-rays is taken over half an hour or so. The radioactive dye shows up white on the X-rays, revealing the structure of the kidneys and urinary tract.

Apart from the hazard of exposure to X-rays, the disadvantage of the procedure is that the dye injected often produces allergic reactions and has even been known to cause death. Both patient and urologist can be grateful for the advent of the modern non-invasive and accurate ultrasound scan.

Two other types of scanning that may be used, particularly if prostate cancer or kidney abnormalities are suspected, are *computed tomography* (CT) *scanning* and *magnetic resonance imaging* (MRI).

In CT scanning, a computer constructs a two-dimensional image of a cross section of the body from data obtained by taking X-rays at 1 cm intervals. As well as providing a cross-sectional view (ordinary X-rays only offer a longitudinal view), CT scanning can show differences in density far better than conventional X-rays.

MRI also uses computer assistance but has the advantage of not exposing the patient to any radiation, and no contrast material, such as barium or radioisotopes, needs to be used. The equipment is extremely expensive and not yet widely available.

Differences between benign and malignant enlargement

Men sometimes suppose that 'benign' enlargement is simply a pre-cancerous condition, and that that is why surgeons sometimes seem so eager to remove it. There is however no evidence of anything of the kind.

In fact, a major difference between the two is that while benign enlargement occurs in the part of the prostate round the urethra and gradually works outward, malignant growth begins in the outer part of the gland (which is why the urologist feels the surface of the gland in the rectal examination to see if he can detect any lumps or irregularities).

Benign enlargement (*benign prostatic hyperplasia* – BPH) is to all intents and purposes a type of benign tumour. It almost universally occurs in middle-aged and elderly men, apparently as part of the ageing process, although it does not always create problems. It is common (though often unrecognized) in all men over 45, and 75 per cent of American men over 50 are estimated to have some symptoms of BPH. Its causes are not fully understood, but the disease is certainly linked in some way with hormonal balance or hormone metabolism.

In fact it is now understood that the 'adenoma', as the tumorous growth is called, is triggered by the presence of dihydrotestosterone, a metabolite of the male hormone. One promising line of research is to attempt to inhibit the production of this substance with a pill (see page 89).

Because prostate cancer starts in the outer cells of the gland, the prostate operation done for benign enlargement will not necessarily prevent the development of cancer in the future, because the outer wall or 'pod' is left intact in the operation.

The causes of prostate cancer are even less well understood

than those of BPH, and it does not seem to be particularly associated with any occupation or activity. Like benign enlargement, however, its progress is dependent on the presence of certain hormones, and removal of the testes (orchidectomy, in medical parlance) is sometimes performed to contain its spread, as the testicles are the main source of the male hormone testosterone, which seems necessary for the proliferation of this cancer.

Neither BPH nor cancer seem to be connected in any way with sexual activity (or the lack of it). Both diseases are found among monks and libertines alike.

Prostatitis

'Prostatitis' is used to describe a whole range of conditions which have in common inflammation or pain, but are not malignant and do not usually create urinary problems. It is very common and, while it can sometimes be cleared up with treatment, often continues as a chronic condition that simply has to be lived with.

It is a complaint mainly of younger men, and is less common in men over 50, unlike BPH or cancer which are rare under that age. Usually it results from an infection of some kind, but occasionally no evidence of infection can be found.

Since the prostate gland has multiple ducts opening onto the urethra, it is clear that any infection in the urine can easily pass up the ducts into the urethra. The internal structure of the prostate is complex, with hundreds of tiny sacs and tubules, and it seems that an infection, once established, can lurk in these crevices and interstices for years, because they are not easily reached by antibiotics circulating in the bloodstream.

The different forms of prostatitis, and their symptoms and treatment, are described in detail in Chapter 6. When prostatitis becomes a chronic complaint, it can flare up time and again, often causing the men affected considerable discomfort and sometimes upsetting their sex lives. For urologists it is a frustrating condition, often resisting medical treatment with remarkable stubbornness.

The patient with prostatitis will only have to undergo a few of the tests mentioned above: probably only a urine analysis and a rectal examination (which may be painful), since the infected prostate usually has a softer, 'boggy' consistency. Another test often required is an analysis of prostatic fluid, produced by massage through the rectum, to help identify the infecting organism.

Not surprisingly, men with prostate problems often suggest that if one were designing a man, one would have not bothered with a prostate – or at least not placed the gland in a place where it could so obviously create trouble. Indeed, the prostate would seem to be one of evolution's failures, a dinosaur of an organ, its original functions largely obsolete and its behaviour deranged by modern man's lifestyle and longevity.

Case history 1.1

Bob T., a driver, used to have to get up two or three times a night 'which I thought was normal at my age of 63'. When he did mention it to his doctor, he was referred to a consultant 'who found nothing much wrong and told me to carry on normally'.

Then he began to have the classic symptoms of hesitancy and urgency. 'One day I was "caught short" but could not make water right away. I was worried but when I got home several hours later I found I was all right again.'

Symptoms became more frequent until 'one morning after getting a rush trip I suddenly had to make water there and then in the car seat.' He went back to his doctor, was referred to a different urologist, and was soon admitted to hospital for a prostate operation.

Case history 1.2

In his late 60s, Paul L. experienced increasing frequency of the need to pass water, 'which was getting more and more of a nuisance. Like for instance: how to space out a car journey from London to, say, the coast – where on the way could I be sure to find a petrol station with a functional "Gents"? I could generally manage about 50 miles without stopping. But also I had to make sure not to start on any journey too soon after breakfast which with me consists mainly of four cups of (real) coffee. Much interrupted nights – every 2–2½ hours. I tried various pills – some homoeopathic – with no results whatsoever.'

Through personal connections, he was referred to a Professor of Urology, who did an IVP X-ray and advised a transurethral operation, although giving Mr L. no information about possible side-effects. 'He did explain to me the technicalities of the transurethral operation, but was quite shocked when I suggested (as I come from a medical background) that he use local anaesthesia and let me watch the operation on a TV monitor (as his pupils do).'

The operation went well – but this was not the end of Mr L.'s problems (see Case history 4.2).

Case history 1.3

In October 1963, the British Prime Minister, Harold Macmillan, resigned after being stricken with acute prostate trouble and faced with an immediate operation. Aged 67, Macmillan was tired and run down, no doubt partly as a result of the urinary obstruction he was suffering.

He had not confided the urinary symptoms he must have had to his private doctor, Sir John Richardson, who could no doubt have rendered the onset of prostate trouble less devastating. When the acute symptoms developed, Sir John was on holiday, and the Prime Minister was seen by a doctor and a urologist who did not know him.

The specialist told him that his symptoms were caused by 'either a benign or a malignant tumour'. Macmillan, a lifelong hypochondriac, immediately assumed the worst, and formed the impression that, at best, he would be laid up for three to four months. By the time that Sir John Richardson had driven down from the Lake District at top speed in his Jaguar, Macmillan had already decided to resign.

According to Macmillan's official biographer, Alistair Horne, both Sir John Richardson and the Prime Minister's son Maurice were convinced that Macmillan resigned unnecessarily in panic at his acute symptoms. Had Sir John known of his symptoms, or been in London when the crisis had occurred, he would almost certainly have been able to reassure the Prime Minister that he would have been back in harness in three to four weeks, not three to four months, and was not as seriously ill as he no doubt felt.

In his memoirs, Macmillan complains how 'this filthy disease' prevented him from attending the Conservative Party Conference, with unfortunate consequences for the Party. He tells how he formally resigned his office while still in hospital: 'Concealed underneath the bed was a pail with a tube full of bile coming out of me. . . I made my resignation to the Queen of England for an hour, in great discomfort.' Alec Douglas-Home became Prime Minister, and Party fortunes declined.

When he was asked on the fateful day by his Press Secretary Harold Evans (later to be Editor of *The Sunday Times* and *The Times*) about the terms of the Press announcement being drafted, Macmillan blurted out: 'Of course I'm finished. I shall probably die.' In fact, like all the best hypochondriacs, he lived to a great age, dying in 1986 in his 93rd year. He never had a recurrence of his prostate trouble, and he always seemed to have regretted his hasty resignation.

CHAPTER 2

Benign enlargement and the development of surgical treatment

Urinary obstruction due to benign enlargement of the prostate has always been a common condition in men over a certain age. In the days before modern surgery it was a dangerous and often fatal complaint, and physicians and surgeons over the centuries have agonized over how to treat it.

It is therefore perhaps surprising that urologists today, as their predecessors for the past 80 or 90 years, have but a single treatment at their disposal when confronted with severe prostatic obstruction: the surgical removal of part or most of the obstructing gland. The operation – prostatectomy – has of course been vastly improved over the years and is now a safe and routine procedure. There are some quite promising less invasive forms of treatment now under trial (see Chapter 5), but their efficacy has yet to be proven, and it seems likely that surgical treatment will remain the standard procedure, for most patients, for many years to come.

Prostatic obstruction has of course become more frequent as life expectancy has increased, for benign enlargement and prostate cancer are both diseases which are much more common in old age than in middle age. So urinary obstruction was not nearly as widely experienced 500 (or even 100) years ago as it is in the rich countries of the world today.

Early methods of treatment

The first medical text mentioning urinary difficulties and obstruction was an Egyptian papyrus of the 15th century BC (now in the Volks-Museum in Leipzig), which also prescribed a medicine for relief of symptoms, concocted from juniper bark, cypress bark and beer. And 1,000 years later in Ancient Greece, Hippocrates recognized the symptoms, if not the cause, and described the outlook for such patients as very poor, noting that the condition was incurable. For 3,000 years, catheterization – the insertion of a tube up the urethra into the bladder to drain it – remained the only effective treatment for urinary retention.

Early catheters were made of different metals (often depending on the status of the patient), and a collection of bronze catheters was recovered from the ruins of Pompeii. Down the ages, catheters were also made from treated paper, wax, gum, elastic, rubber and finally plastic. Catheterization often resulted in infection, and its success as a treatment must have been very limited. Otherwise, early surgeons restricted their intervention to removing bladder stones, which can occur when the bladder does not empty completely because of outflow obstruction.

Drastic remedies

The role of the enlarged prostate in urinary obstruction was understood by the end of the 18th century, and occasionally surgeons had cut away bits of enlarged prostate while operating to remove bladder stones. Alternatives to catheterization which were tried over the centuries included the administration of hemlock and ergot, prostatic massage, vasectomy and even castration. The theory justifying castration was that the prostate failed to grow in young male animals following castration, but it was later shown that castration after the age of 40 does not always reverse benign enlargement (although it does often slow the growth of prostate cancer – see Chapter 8). Despite claims of real improvement made by a Victorian surgeon who specialized in the operation, the procedure did not prove popular.

Early prostate operations

In 1874 the Italian surgeon Enrico Bottini introduced his 'galvanocautery incisor', which was the greatest innovation until the development of the prostatic resector by Hugh Hampton Young, the father of modern urology. But the successful removal of the enlarged gland was not carried out before the late 1880s, when a British surgeon, McGill in Leeds, and two Americans, Belfield of Chicago and Fuller of New York, all described prostatectomy operations.

These early operations were of course fairly crude 'open' abdominal operations, and carried such a high mortality that few were performed, and only in a few hospitals. At the turn of the century, there were still only two common treatments for severe obstruction – self-catheterization and vasectomy.

'Catheter schooling'

The most usual treatment was to admit the patient to hospital for a few days for 'catheter schooling', to train him how to pass a catheter – a thin rubber tube – up his urethra to relieve himself three or four times a day. In the country, the man was often taught at home by his GP. This undoubtedly prolonged life in some cases, but it carried a very high mortality – upwards of 20 per cent of the men dying within the first six months, mainly from infections leading to kidney failure. These men – they would all have been well-off patients to receive such treatment – would carry their catheters and lubricant on their person, or even coiled within the band of their top-hats, for when they were 'taken short'.

Vasectomy

Vasectomy is one of the curiosities of early prostate treatment, since there seems no way that it can ever have had the slightest effect on prostate enlargement.

Vasectomy is of course the cutting and tying of the two vasa deferentia, the tubes which carry sperm from the testicles to the semen ducts. Nowadays, the simple operation is routinely performed as a method of male sterilization, and is believed not to have any side-effects (although some studies have suggested that it is associated with higher rates of prostate can-cer). The only possible way that vasectomy can have affected the prostate was if the surgeon had mistakenly severed the artery serving the testicle as well as the vas. This would have led to testicular atrophy and a lower level of testosterone, which might have had a shrinking effect on a benign or cancerous enlargement.

Nevertheless, at the turn of the century vasectomy was the next most popular treatment for prostatic obstruction after catheter schooling. In fact, John Thomas, the birdkeeper at St James's Park, London, who was the first man to have his prostate removed by Peter Freyer (see below), had already been given bilateral vasectomy to no avail.

Vasectomy used to be carried out routinely before a prostate operation to prevent the spread of any infection to the epididymis, the coiled tubes adjoining the testicles in which the sperm mature and begin their journey up the vas. The operation still tends to be done in some European countries, but not usually in Britain or the United States. Epididymitis is a rare complication of prostate surgery, even in the absence of vasectomy.

The 'open' operations

Credit for popularizing the prostate operation by making it simple, safe and effective usually goes to Sir Peter Freyer of St Peter's Hospital in Covent Garden, London. Freyer's operation, first described in 1901, was the 'suprapubic' operation in which an incision is made through the bladder and the prostate tissue is 'enucleated' (medical jargon for 'shelled out') by the surgeon's finger. Bleeding was often a problem, but the operation had far lower morbidity and mortality rates than any previously attempted, and 'a dangerous surgical adventure became a routine operation'.

This operation remained the standard approach for 40 years, until an Irish surgeon, Terence Millin, described his 'retropubic' operation in 1945, which approached the prostate not through the bladder, but behind the pubic bone and through the prostate capsule. It was quicker, there was less bleeding, and led to a quicker recovery. It is still the operation of choice today if the transurethral approach is not suitable for one reason or another (see below and Chapter 3).

Another type of open operation is that done by the perineal approach, in which the prostate is removed through an incision between the anus and the scrotum. The operation was popular between the wars because of its advantages for the

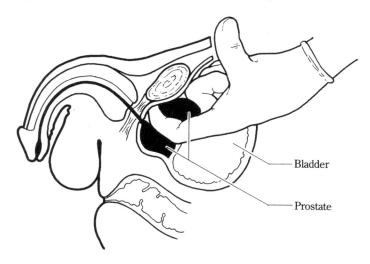

Fig. 2.1: enucleation with surgeon's finger

surgeon, but is rarely done nowadays because it often caused damage to nerves which resulted in impotence.

So open prostate operations became common in the years between the two World Wars, but there was still a relatively high mortality rate of 5 to 15 per cent. It was about this time that endoscopic surgery through the urethra – that is surgery carried out by a special cauterizing instrument which allowed the surgeon direct vision of what he was doing – became a practical possibility.

The transurethral operation

The transurethral, or endoscopic, operation is the operation most commonly done on the prostate today. While it is not true to call it a bloodless operation, since the prostate tissue is richly supplied with blood vessels which bleed when cut into, there is less bleeding than in an abdominal operation and of course no visible scar.

The operation is more fully described in Chapter 3, but briefly surgery is carried out through a resectoscope (see Fig. 3.1) containing a fibre optic light source and a telescope which enables the surgeon to see what tissue he is removing. The 'blade' is a high-frequency electric arc which cuts through the tissue and cauterizes simultaneously. The tissue removed is washed into the bladder by a non-conducting irrigating solution such as glycine, and then removed through a catheter.

The name given to the operation, 'prostatectomy', is actually a misnomer, since it implies removal of the whole of the prostate. Such an operation, sometimes done to treat prostate cancer (see Chapter 8), is known as 'radical prostatectomy'. In it, the whole prostate capsule, together with the seminal vesicles, are removed through an incision in the perineum, and the bladder is joined up directly to the external sphincter. It is a much more difficult and unpleasant operation than transurethral resection (TUR).

In TUR, only the internal prostate tissue is removed, usually down to the capsule; the capsule then shrinks to act as part of the urethra.

As early as the 16th century, a French surgeon, Ambroise Paré, had devised an instrument with a cutting edge which he inserted in the urethra and twisted it back and forth to cut away the 'carnosities' of the prostate. Done blind, this was a hit-and-miss and dangerous operation, and few surgeons attempted it. In the 19th century there was renewed interest in the transurethral approach, and an Italian surgeon, Enrico Bottini of Pavia, invented a cauterizing instrument with a platinum element designed to burn prostatic tissue.

The Bottini instrument was also blind, but was modified in 1900 by the incorporation of an optical system. The first proper TURs were done in 1927 in the Mayo Clinic in Minnesota, by Bumpus and Thompson. But it was not until 1932, when the McCarthy direct-vision resectoscope was perfected, that transurethral surgery became popular and safe. When the first mortality figures were published for transurethral resection, as the new prostate operation was called, they were greeted with disbelief by the surgical establishment.

McCarthy's instrument, refined and improved in various ways over the years, became the resectoscope used by surgeons today all over the world. Its popularity grew rapidly in the United States, and by 1945 transurethral resection was the standard procedure there for treating prostatic obstruction.

A final improvement to the resectoscope was made in the 1970s: this was the design of a continuous irrigation system. It has two advantages: the field of view is kept clear, and the pressure inside the bladder is kept low. Keeping the pressure of the irrigating fluid in the bladder low may help to avoid the 'TUR syndrome', caused by fluid entering the patient's venous system during a long operation. This so-called Iglesias system (named after its Spanish inventor) relies on a free return of fluid through multiple openings in the outer sheath of the resectoscope.

But despite its popularity in the United States, TUR took far longer to become established in Britain and Europe generally.

Writing in the first British standard work on the subject, *Transurethral Resection*, published in 1971, John Blandy wrote that 'the prevailing climate of surgical opinion is still against transurethral resection'. And as late as 1978, in another book, Blandy reported that as many as 80 per cent of prostatectomies in Britain were still performed by open routes.

Since TUR was clearly a much safer operation, with lower mortality and morbidity and a shorter hospital stay, what accounted for the reluctance of the British surgical establishment? The real objection, according to Blandy, was that the operation is 'hard to learn and hard to teach'. It is a more delicate operation than open abdominal surgery, and it cannot be learnt by students looking over a great surgeon's shoulder.

Today, students may watch the procedure on a video screen, but there are still few other operations like it in the demands made on the surgeon. 'Even today,' Professor Blandy writes, 'no operation makes such demands on his concentration; there are no slack periods during a transurethral resection when one can relax and allow an assistant to finish a suture line or close a wound. From the moment the resectoscope slides into the prostatic cavity, his attention must never waver.'

Variations in the operation

In the early days in the United States, surgeons often tended to remove only the 'adenoma' (the enlarged part of the gland), leaving the normal part behind. But it was found that in these cases the adenoma grew back more quickly, necessitating a further operation, and it is now standard practice, both in Britain and the United States, to remove the prostate tissue down to the capsule.

However, it is still the case that the weight of tissue removed in TURs in the United States is under half that removed in operations in Britain. This may well be because American urologists tend to intervene earlier, and US medicine may be better generally at early diagnosis. This is borne out by the fact that a far larger proportion of men over 60 – some 30 per cent as against 10 per cent in Britain – have a TUR.

An exception to the rule that all prostate tissue is removed is that, in some cases, surgeons find they can get away with carrying out what is called a resection of the bladder neck. Normally in benign enlargement, as well as mechanical obstruction of the urethra by the glandular enlargement (adenoma), there is some swelling, or hypertrophy, of the exit of the bladder (bladder neck), which may cause as much, or more, obstruction to the urine outflow as the enlargement of the prostate itself. When it is clear that the bladder neck hypertrophy is the main cause of the problem, the urologist may prefer to remove sufficient tissue from the bladder neck, and not resect the whole of the prostate gland – or even just make an incision to widen the bladder exit. The operation is shorter, but it does not always do the trick, and often a complete resection of the prostate has to be done a few years later.

Other forms of transurethral operation

Although the endoscopic resectoscope is by far and away the most commonly used instrument for carrying out prostatectomies, there are other techniques which are sometimes used, and are worth briefly describing.

One instrument, used for early transurethral operations and still popular with a few American surgeons, is the cold punch. This uses a circular hollow knife, instead of a cauterizing arc, to remove the prostate tissue. The instrument has a bright light source, enabling the surgeon to see what he is doing, but does not use irrigating solution: the excised tissue passes back through the tube of the instrument. Any bleeding is controlled by electrocoagulation by a standard resectoscope, which may indeed be used to finish off the nooks and crannies difficult to reach with the punch. One big advantage of the cold punch is its speed: it is much quicker to cut away tissue with a knife than with a 'hot loop'.

Another method of removing prostate tissue through the urethra is laser surgery. Here the tissue is simply vaporized by the intense heat of the laser beam. Attractive in theory, the procedure has proved to have several drawbacks in practice, and is now rarely used. Lasers are however employed successfully in urology for shattering stones in the ureters, and in treating cancer of the prostate and bladder. They are also used experimentally in another way for shrinking, rather than destroying, prostate tissue (see Chapter 6).

An unusual procedure which has the advantages of being able to be carried out quickly and with only local anaesthesia, is *cryosurgery* (see Fig. 2.2), which is surgery by freezing. This is based on the principle that a copper element supercooled with liquid nitrogen will create an ice-ball of a certain size and shape (see Fig. 2.3).

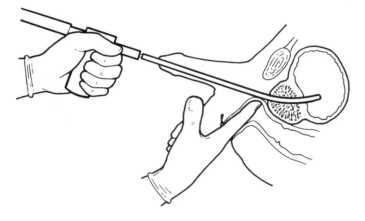

Fig. 2.2: cryosurgery

In this operation, a specially designed probe, with a copper element which can be cooled by circulating liquid nitrogen and electrically reheated, is inserted in the urethra and accurately sited in the prostate by means of a reference knob which can be felt by the surgeon's finger in the rectum. The temperature is lowered first to 0°C, then to –40°C, then if all is well, to –160°C. The surgeon then monitors the formation of the ice-ball with a finger in the patient's rectum. After about five to ten minutes, depending on the size of the prostate, the probe is warmed and removed.

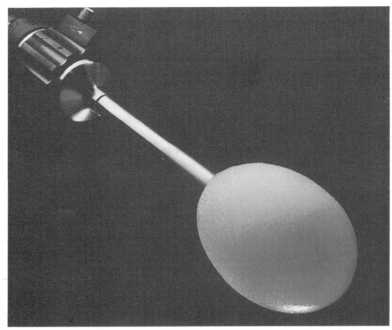

Photograph courtesy of Spembly

Fig. 2.3: ice-ball

The deep-frozen tissue shrinks as water is absorbed into the ice-ball, and is flushed out through the catheter. There is a little bleeding, but the freezing front of the ice-ball effectively cauterizes most of it. The patient does not need general anaesthesia and suffers little discomfort. But the procedure is skilled and is not widely available. Its proponents believe it is useful for patients in poor health who would be unable to undergo a TUR, and claim that, in skilled hands, cryosurgery can have results as good as TUR.

One possible future development which may make the transurethral operation much quicker, and so safer for the patient, is *robotic surgery* – surgery carried out with the help of a robot. The TUR operation is unlike most others in that it involves a long series of repetitive movements to cut away the enlarged tissues in hundreds of 'slices'. Computer-assisted robots are very good at performing repetitive tasks very accurately.

Urologists at St Peter's Hospital, London, have collaborated with scientists at Imperial College on a feasibility study in which a robot helps the surgeon by carrying out the task of cutting away the tissue under the surgeon's supervision. Substituting a potato for the prostate, they set up a robot, consisting of a cutter on a drive shaft attached to a six-axis machine and a high-speed motor.

A video camera was attached to the instrument, permitting a visual display of the cutting process and allowing the surgeon to monitor it. In a fraction of the time taken by a surgeon using a resectoscope – five minutes as opposed to at least an hour – the robot produced a perfectly clear cut in the potato. Instead of using the usual electrical arc knife, the robot used a metal blade, similar to that of a kitchen blender, capable of rotating at 40,000 rpm. The robot also has an excellent understanding of three dimensions, whereas surgeons do not always possess perfect spatial skills and often have to go back to the initial position during an operation to reorientate themselves.

The robot is now being tried out on cadaver prostates, but it will probably be at least five years before robots are available to help the urological surgeon. Once they have got used to the idea, most surgeons will probably welcome the assistance of a robot. Many of them end up with chronic neck-ache and back-ache from continuously peering down the endoscope, often at awkward angles. Using a robot, the surgeon would sit at a visual display unit watching the view as if from inside the prostate.

'The main advantage of the technique,' according to John Wickham, Director of the London Institute of Urology, who is in charge of the project, 'is speed. It would shorten the operation dramatically. In five minutes, the robot, guided by ultrasound, would remove the necessary tissue according to a pre-arranged, tailor-made, pattern, then the surgeon would go in with his hot wire to cauterize the bleeding veins.'

The use of a robot in surgical operations is illegal at present, and there is some way to go in developing failsafe software for the robot before anyone could suggest that the law is changed. But in the long run, it does seem a likely prospect that robots will be enlisted to help with prostatic surgery, and this could help reduce waiting lists for prostate operations – although new non-surgical treatments may make an impact before the robot is perfected (see Chapter 5).

TUR under local anaesthetic

Two groups of surgeons, one in the UK and one in the United States, are carrying out transurethral prostatectomies under local anaesthetic. Prostatectomies have been done under epidural – spinal – anaesthesia for many years: this makes the whole of the lower part of the body numb, but it is complicated and slightly risky to administer and is not suitable for patients with heart trouble. In this new procedure, the lower part of the bladder and the nerves serving the prostate itself are blocked by local anaesthesia delivered through the urethra.

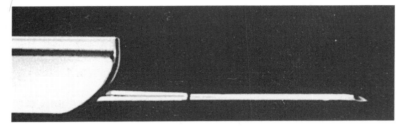

Photograph courtesy of *World Journal of Urology* No. 361

Fig. 2.4: endoneedle

The patient is given a tranquillizing injection of Midazolam, which makes him relaxed and drowsy. After anaesthetizing the urethra with anaesthetic gel squeezed up through the penis, the surgeon then uses a specially designed hypodermic needle which is passed through the endoscope up the urethra to inject lignocaine, a local anaesthetic, into the base of the bladder and the prostate itself. The surgeon then carries out a standard TUR or bladder neck incision, as appropriate. The procedure is most suitable for prostates that are not too large – the maximum weight of tissue removed is around 40g, which is above the average. This is because the tranquillizer and local anaesthetic wear off after a time, and the patient may also develop cramps if he is elderly, so the surgeon has to finish his work quickly (although the patient can always be 'topped up' with intravenous tranquillizer). At least 60 per cent of prostates are suitable for this method.

'We treat the prostate cavity like a dentist treats the mouth,' says Mr Ron Miller, surgeon in charge of the team at the Royal Northern Hospital, London. The whole procedure is over within 30 minutes. The patients are usually home within 36 hours, and do very well. What is more, the patients seem to prefer the procedure, and certainly do not find it particularly unpleasant or painful. The new technique dispenses with saline drips and lengthy catheterization.

'We have done over 300 patients and trained a number of urologists in the technique, but many people in the profession still refuse to believe that it's possible,' says Mr Miller. 'But probably within four or five years, most TURs will be done this way.'

Indications for open surgery

Finally, there are certain groups of patients for whom the transurethral approach is not suitable, and who must, if surgery is inevitable, therefore undergo an 'open' prostatectomy (through an abdominal incision).

Very large prostates are usually removed by open surgery for two reasons: firstly it takes time to remove tissue by TUR, and a surgeon may not want to carry out a very long operation, especially on an elderly and/or infirm patient; and secondly, a large prostate may be so long that the prostatic urethra is prolonged into the bladder and the endoscope is unable to reach the bladder neck. The usual weight of an enlarged prostate is 20–30 g; if it is over 70–80g, then the surgeon must consider an open procedure. Only 5 or 10 per cent of cases fall into this category.

Another group of patients who may require open surgery are those men with osteoarthritis of the hip joints, not an uncommon condition in the elderly. This is because the stiffness of the joints makes it impossible to position the patient correctly for TUR (with his knees up and apart). Sometimes a TUR can be performed with difficulty, by raising the operating table as high as possible with the surgeon performing the resection below the patient's legs, but usually the surgeon will prefer to do an open operation.

Many prostate patients have associated bladder problems. If there are bladder stones, these can usually be dealt with by litholapaxy (crushing by an instrument inserted transurethrally), unless they are huge (over 10cm or 4 inches), in which case an open prostatectomy may be required. If there are diverticula (blow-outs) which require surgical removal, then it will be best to remove the prostate through an incision in the bladder (suprapubic or transvesical operation).

CHAPTER 3

Having a prostatectomy

Once your prostate problem has been assessed by your urologist, he will discuss treatment with you. At present, the only effective treatment available for urinary outflow caused by benign enlargement is a prostatectomy – that is, removal of the enlarged tissue of the prostate gland. Some new treatments are now on trial (see Chapter 5), but it will be some time before these are available for most people.

This chapter will look at what you should expect if you have a prostatectomy, how the operation is performed, what will happen after the operation and how you can help yourself to make the procedure as untraumatic as possible.

Talking to your doctor

Men often find it hard to discuss personal matters with anyone, including their doctor. They may feel very threatened at the prospect of being examined intimately and having to discuss things about which there is a taboo in our culture – excretion and sexuality. However, it can be very important to be able to talk about these matters openly – not only will this help your doctor or urologist understand how severe your condition is, and whether you really need an operation, but will also help to put your mind at rest and remove unnecessary fears.

Seeing your urologist, especially for the first time, can be a very difficult encounter. You may have had to wait weeks or months for the appointment, and then find yourself waiting with other anxious-looking men in an overcrowded clinic. Your urologist, when you meet him, may seem busy and offhand. It can be very difficult in these circumstances to have a meaningful discussion with him, or to ask the questions you want.

It may help to write down the essential questions to which you seek answers. If you don't understand the reply fully, say so. 'I'm afraid I didn't quite catch the last bit,' or, 'You used a medical term I didn't understand there – could you put that into ordinary English?' will do nicely.

Try not to let yourself be hustled out of the room without getting the answers you need. Ask direct questions about how long you will be laid up, and what possible side-effects the operation may have. Make sure that it really is necessary to your health that you have the operation – some men may find that their symptoms are not severe enough to warrant an operation now and surgery always has its risks (see Chapter 4).

Many urologists are so used to dealing with prostate problems that they forget that the men they see may be deeply embarrassed, ashamed of the way their bodies have let them down, and fearful about the effect the operation may have on them. If prostate cancer is suspected, men may fear truly terrible consequences: drastic surgery to remove the whole prostate gland, possibly removal of the testes if the cancer has spread to prevent its growth, and possible death.

The prostate as part of a man's sexual apparatus is the cause of many deep-seated anxieties, and it is important to raise your fears even if the urologist seems dismissive of them. It is your body and your right to know what will be done to it.

Many doctors will respect a patient who wants to know about the operation and is likely to volunteer more information to him than someone who sits quietly and nods 'yes' to everything. There are some other 'tricks' you can learn to help get the most out of your doctor. Firstly, shaking hands confidently and introducing yourself when you enter the urologist's consulting room makes a completely different impression from the man who creeps in and waits meekly to be spoken to.

If you are admitted to hospital and will see the urologist before any tests or action is taken, don't immediately get undressed and into bed. Sit fully dressed by the bed and read your book or chat to other patients. It has been shown that doctors treat people differently when they are in bed in pyjamas from how they deal with fully-dressed people who are up and about.

Effect on sexuality

This is one of men's major fears on seeking a urologist and contemplating the prospect of a prostatectomy. The prospect of having a sexual organ tampered with in any way is very threatening, and most men fear that their sex lives may be affected. Many men are so afraid of this outcome that they cannot even raise it with their urologist, and therefore continue to be afraid; this fear may itself affect their sexual lives afterwards. A man who expects to be made impotent or have his sexual drive reduced after the operation may well find that stress and anxiety about his sexual performance create these very problems.

Men who are to have a prostatectomy should ask and be reassured that there will be no effect on their sexual desire or performance, though it is important that they should also be told that it is likely that they will be infertile following the operation.

Many doctors seem embarrassed at discussing sexuality with their patients, and many patients are probably embarrassed too, so it is not surprising that often men leave the consulting room without discussing the matter fully or seeking the reassurance they need. Many doctors will dismiss any query the man has with a swift assertion that the operation 'has no effect on sexuality'. This is not always honest, as this man explains:

> I was reassured by my doctor saying this, as I had a young wife and two small children. However my wife, who wanted another baby, was not so easily reassured and looked at a medical book in the library. Here she read that a prostatectomy frequently led to infertility, because the sperm are ejaculated backwards into the bladder at orgasm. I admit I was horrified at not being told. One's fertility is a fundamental part of sexuality, and how dare a doctor assume that just because you were 'old enough' to need prostate surgery you were too old to want to father a child?

Many men do not find out about this side-effect until they sign the consent forms for the operation, by which time they are hardly in a position to remonstrate. One 70-year-old man was told: 'By the way, you won't be able to have any more children,' as he was prepared for surgery. Many men are not adequately forewarned about retrograde ejaculation, which may distress them when it occurs after the operation. At least being told in advance gives someone a chance to become reconciled to the fact before agreeing to the operation so that he feels he has consented to it.

Partial information is almost as bad as no information. The 70-year-old told that he won't be able to have any more children will probably have no plans whatsoever for fathering more children, but may become distressed because he believes he is really being told, 'You won't be able to have any more sex.' It is also common sense (and proved by several studies) that men who are given full explanations as to the nature of the operation and its likely side-effects are far less likely to have sexual problems afterwards than men who were told little or nothing.

The idea that prostatectomy can cause impotence or other sexual problems has been responsible for making many men conceal their symptoms till the last possible moment. Partly this fear arises from lingering 'folk memories' of the old perineal prostate operation (hardly ever performed today) or the radical prostatectomy, in which the whole prostate, capsule and all, is removed (sometimes performed for prostate cancer): in both these operations the nerves supplying the penis were often severed, leading to impotence. When these operations are done nowadays it is usually possible to avoid cutting these nerves.

Occasionally psychological impotence can follow the operation, especially if the man is very afraid that this might happen; if so, help from a counsellor or sex therapist or an understanding partner can help.

There is an unfortunate attitude among many urologists that their prostate patients are really 'too old' to be interested in sex. They may have an unrealistic attitude to men's sexual lives. One West German book for the general reader confidently asserts that 'fewer than 10 per cent of men over 60 have normal sexual potency (defined as having sexual intercourse without difficulty at least once a month)'. One wonders what men were surveyed to provide evidence for this extraordinary claim.

With divorce and remarriage becoming much more common, many men today have younger wives and may be having second families, and it is known for men to be sexually active and father children well into old age. There really is no excuse for not treating men's fears about loss of part of their sexual lives seriously.

The possibility of retrograde ejaculation, even if a man is not concerned about his fertility, may still be distressing to some couples, and a urologist is unlikely to be able to deal with this. To some men or their wives, the idea of sperm and semen being ejaculated into the bladder is simply 'not nice'. Just as women may regret the loss of their womb after hysterectomy even if they were well beyond childbearing, men may regret the loss of the potential to be a father. It is a pity that both men themselves and their doctors are not more able to discuss these matters openly to help men come to terms with feelings of fear and loss

Doctors are fond of pointing out that there are some elderly men who do not lead very active sex lives because they or their wives are no longer interested, and some who lose interest in sex after a major operation, but the modern prostate operation should not be a greater risk factor than any abdominal operation. A man might even use a prostate operation as an excuse for not having sex which he had really ceased to enjoy with his partner. If a man is otherwise healthy after the operation and has a stable relationship with a loving partner, there is no reason why his sex life should be in any way affected, and he can really forget any fear of impotence.

Modern techniques of prostatectomy

The operation that is almost always performed today is known as TUR – transurethral prostatectomy. The operation is carried out by introducing an instrument through the urethra and cutting away at the enlarged prostate tissue. Because there is no cut in the abdominal wall some people imagine that this is not a 'proper' operation, but this is of course not the case.

A TUR is a fairly major operation, requiring up to a week's stay in hospital. If a man is healthy and all is well, he can be expected to go home as little as five days after the operation; if he is unwell, or has complications following the operation such as an infection, he might have to stay in longer.

Before the operation, the hospital will carry out tests to ensure no infection is present in the urine, and blood analysis to check whether the kidneys are functioning normally.

If you do have a urinary tract infection, the operation will normally be postponed for a few days while antibiotics are given and the infection clears up, because no surgeon likes to operate when an infection is present unless it is absolutely necessary.

If the blood tests show that there is too much urea and creatinine in the blood, this means that your kidneys are not functioning properly because of back pressure from the bladder (a condition called *hydronephrosis*). A catheter will then be inserted to drain your bladder, and the operation is likely to be postponed for 10 to 14 days while your kidneys recover from the stress of hydronephrosis. You will be sent home with an 'indwelling catheter' which drains into a bag strapped to your thigh – not as bad as it sounds once you get used to it. Experience has shown that men whose kidneys are not under strain recover much better from the operation.

The urologist may also ask for an ultrasound scan to be made of your bladder, and sometimes may wish to do a cystoscopy. (Both these procedures are described in Chapter 1). Normally, the cystoscopy is done immediately before the operation while you are already under the anaesthetic.

The transurethral operation is carried out with an instrument known as a resectoscope (see Fig. 3.1). The most com-

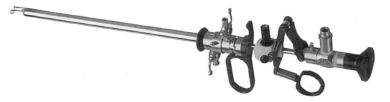

Photograph courtesy of Karl Storz GmbH & Co.

Fig. 3.1: resectoscope

mon kind uses an electric current to cut away the prostate tissue, while the other kind uses a tubular knife-blade. The urologist is able to see what he is doing by viewing along a fibre optic cable.

The surgeon trims away the prostate tissue from the inside

towards the outside. The new growth in the prostate occurs in the centre, and so the operation removes this tissue, working back to the original prostate tissue. It is rather like inserting a knife into the core of an apple and removing the flesh from the inside back towards the skin till all the core is removed. Depending on whether the middle or lateral lobes of the prostate are enlarged, differing amounts of tissue may need to be removed; if the middle lobe is enlarged, only a small amount of tissue may need to be removed, while with enlargement of the lateral lobes it tends to be much greater.

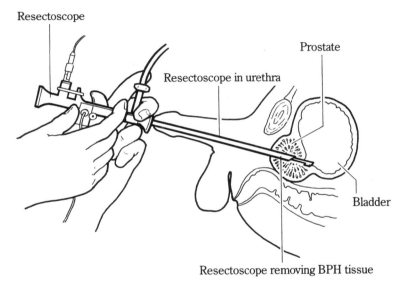

Fig. 3.2: tissue being removed with resectoscope

Unfortunately, many blood vessels have to be cut in the course of the operation, and unlike in an open operation, they cannot be tied off before cutting because of the urologist's limited view through the resectoscope. The bladder therefore needs to be washed out with fluid during the operation to wash away the blood and enable the urologist to see what he is doing. The bleeding blood vessels are coagulated or 'cooked' with electrical current to seal them off as the operation continues. The pieces of prostate tissue which have been removed are also washed away with the irrigating fluid.

The TUR is clearly a difficult procedure to carry out and

requires a skilled urologist. He needs to remove all the obstructing prostate tissue and sometimes the normal tissue as well, stop blood vessels bleeding too much as they are cut, and must take care not to damage the bladder neck or sphincter, as doing so could result in incontinence. The operation is therefore carried out only by skilled urologists and not by ordinary general surgeons. However, new doctors do need to train and will do so supervised by a skilled urologist. You might prefer not to be used for training someone, and it is perfectly within your rights to ask who will be performing the operation, and to ask whether it can be the consultant himself rather than a more junior doctor or trainee.

The operation can be quite a long one – on average about one to one-and-a-half hours – and can be done either under general anaesthetic or with an epidural. The latter is an injection of anaesthetic into the epidural space in the spine between the vertebrae and the membrane enclosing the spinal cord. You will be asked to lie on your side and curl up as much as possible to make it easier for the anaesthetist to put the needle into the spine. A local anaesthetic prevents you feeling the tube go in; you feel the anaesthetic being put in like a cold fluid running down your legs. A catheter is left in your back so that the epidural can be 'topped up.' You will also be given some kind of tranquillizer to relax you during the operation.

You will be unable to feel anything in the lower part of your body while the epidural is working. The epidural also takes some time to wear off, offering pain relief for some time after the operation. It does not carry many of the risks of a general anaesthetic, especially to the lungs, and is often used for older patients.

After the operation

If you have a general anaesthetic, you will probably wake from the operation feeling groggy and perhaps sick. You will find yourself wired up to an alarming number of tubes and drips. A Foley catheter will have been inserted into the urethra at the end of the operation – this is held in place by a balloon which is inflated inside the bladder to prevent the catheter slipping out. The catheter is left in place for several days until the small blood vessels which have not been sealed off during surgery have sealed themselves and stopped bleeding.

Nowadays the bladder is usually continuously irrigated with a saline solution for a day or two after surgery to minimize the chances of clots forming in the bladder, which can cause painful spasms of the bladder and prevent urine draining, and this means more bags of fluid and tubes hanging round the bed.

After 24 hours you will usually have all these tubes and bags removed except for the catheter and drainage bag; you should be able to eat and drink and move around, taking the drainage bag with you, which is usually attached to a little stand. The urine will usually change colour, as one urologist put it, from 'a rich claret through rosé to something approaching normal'. You will be advised to drink a lot of fluid – six pints a day – to wash out the bladder and help prevent clots and also to reduce the discomfort.

One thing which a surgeon always does after a prostate operation is to examine the tissue removed for signs of latent cancer. He will tell you a day or two after the operation what the result is. Usually, nothing is found – and sometimes the puzzled patient is told just this (see Introduction). Unsuspected latent cancer is found in about 5 per cent of TUR patients.

If cancer cells are found, this is not necessarily a cause for great concern, as some presence of cancer cells in the prostate is quite common in older men. You should try to find out from your surgeon what degree of cancer presence was found. It may be a case of having some radiation or chemotherapy treatment there and then, 'just to be on the safe side', or you may be asked to undergo scanning or other tests to establish whether the cancer has spread outside the prostate. Unless the possibility of cancer was mentioned to you before the operation, because the urologist detected cancer-like nodules during the rectal examination, this is unlikely. (See Chapter 8.)

Normally pain or discomfort are not great following a TUR and pain relief following the operation will usually be offered, but is often not necessary.

If you have had an open operation rather than a TUR, you will certainly be in some pain after the operation – from the abdominal wound, not from the prostate itself. You will probably have had the retropubic operation (see Chapter 2), which involves a long incision below the navel. Or you may have had the suprapubic or transvesical operation, in which the prostate tissue is removed through the bladder; in this case you will have a drainage tube in your lower abdomen as well as a catheter for a few days.

Your recovery will be slower than a man who has had a TUR, because there is more tissue healing to take place, and you may need to stay in hospital for 10–14 days. But when you have fully recovered, the effects will be the same.

When you go home

You will be advised to rest when you go home after the operation and not to work or undertake any strenuous physical activity for a while, usually four weeks, just in case a scab comes away from a blood vessel prematurely and results in renewed bleeding. Any bleeding following the operation should be reported to your doctor.

Although, depending on your previous symptoms, immediate relief may follow a prostatectomy, in that you will not experience difficulty in passing urine, you may find that it takes some time for things to settle down. At first you may still need to pass water frequently, especially if advised to continue drinking more fluids than normal, and you may still find urgency a problem and not be able to hold on for long once you feel you need to pee. You may find too that you still get up in the night to pee, though this may be more from habit than necessity, and you will probably gradually adjust so you no longer need to get up at night, or at least not more than once.

If the bladder has been stretched and weakened by years of trying to force urine out and ultimately lost the battle, it may take some time for it to return to something like its normal tone; in some cases it may never do so. If the bladder has been overstretched, it may never be able to expel urine with the force it once did, and the flow rate may not be greatly improved, even if there is no more obstruction and the bladder is completely emptied.

However, most men will find a great improvement in their flow rate – perhaps as much as 200 per cent, say from 5 ml per second to 20 ml per second – sometimes within days of the operation, sometimes with a gradual improvement over weeks or months. The stream no longer ends up in a miserable dribble, but cuts off cleanly. You no longer have to lean right over the toilet bowl to avoid wetting the floor.

Urgency and frequency will lessen too, and the capacity of your bladder will improve – not of course to what it used to be when you were in your 20s or 30s, but at least so that you no longer suffer social inconvenience, or have to be always on the lookout for a public lavatory.

Getting up at night may continue to be a bit of a problem for some men, especially if you are over 70. This is because, in the elderly, the normal pattern of urine production is changed, with as much or more being produced during the night hours as during the day. This may mean that you will have to get up once or twice during the night – but this happens to older women too. And now, when you do need to go, you do actually pass a substantial volume of urine, not just a feeble trickle as often happened before.

CHAPTER 4

Limitations and side-effects of prostatectomy

The modern transurethral prostate operation is an extremely successful procedure. Most men recover from it well, are completely cured of their urinary obstruction, their bladder returns more or less to normal, and their sexual performance is essentially unaffected.

From the surgeon's point of view, it is a demanding but satisfying procedure, a specialized operation using delicate high-technology equipment; mortality in his mainly elderly patients is well under 1 per cent, and most of them are out of hospital in five days and performing normally within a month. It is, undoubtedly, a vast improvement on the early prostate operations, which involved much higher mortality, greater loss of blood and risk of infection and a normal hospital stay of at least two weeks.

In short, as a leading British urologist put it, the TUR operation for benign enlargement is 'the Gold Standard against which we must judge the success of all new alternative treatments'.

However, the operation does have its side-effects, drawbacks and limitations, and it is as well to be aware of these.

Retrograde ejaculation

The most common side-effect is retrograde ejaculation, already described in Chapter 3. Its incidence after the operation has been reported to vary between 30 and 90 per cent. It does seem to occur rather less frequently with TUR than with open surgery. If the operation is carried out thoroughly, it should theoretically always occur, and the reasons for its occurrence or non-occurrence are not entirely clear. It probably depends on how much tissue from the bladder neck has been removed during the operation: if the bladder neck sphincter is still capable of closing, then ejaculation will still occur normally.

Sometimes retrograde ejaculation is not total, or does not totally occur every time; for this reason it is unwise to rely on it as a form of contraception. Drugs have been successfully used to help the bladder neck contract: alpha-sympathetic agents (which work in the opposite way to the alpha-blockers used to improve voiding in prostate patients – see Chapter 5) such as ephedrine, neosynephrine and phenylpropanolamine have had good results in some men, and if concerned, you should ask your doctor if you can try them.

Many urologists claim that retrograde ejaculation makes no difference to the sensation of orgasm. Since orgasm is highly subjective, this is surely a rash claim: a more honest appreciation is that the sensation is 'different, but acceptable'. The feeling of semen being forced through the urethra is clearly going to be missing, and some female partners, even if they are not interested in getting pregnant, are disappointed by the 'dry climax'.

In fact a study carried out in 1982 found that over 30 per cent even of those men who were still able to ejaculate after the operation experienced a decrease or change in the character of orgasm. And of those (the majority) who had retrograde ejaculation, 70 per cent experienced a decrease or change in intensity of orgasm.

As mentioned in Chapter 3, many urologists underestimate the importance that, rightly or wrongly, men usually attach to the ability to ejaculate. Writing in a recently published book for the general reader, one American urologist confessed: 'As a general rule, almost all patients undergoing surgery for BPH are beyond the age where fatherhood is of interest to them, but it is *absolutely amazing* to me that many patients are *extremely annoyed*, and even angry, when they find that they have retrograde ejaculation *unless they have been forewarned of this*.' [my italics]

A man with a younger wife may well want to have more children, and in this case retrograde ejaculation is more than a mere disappointment. This situation makes such a man a prime candidate for some other form of treatment which does not affect fertility, and he should press his urologist to try non-surgical treatment.

Should this approach fail and surgery be inevitable, the man should then consider banking his sperm. In Britain, for some unexplained reason, this service is not available on the National Health Service, but it can be arranged quite inexpensively through a medical charity, the British Pregnancy Advisory Service. In the United States, most urologists can arrange the service.

The process of preserving sperm by freezing for later insemination has of course been understood for years, and much of today's livestock is produced by artificial insemination with frozen semen. Specimens of semen are usually produced by masturbation but special condoms (without spermicide) can be provided to collect the semen during normal intercourse. The semen must be delivered to the laboratory within an hour or so of ejaculation, and kept warm in the meantime.

On the first occasion, the technician checks that the sperm is normal and can survive deep-freezing. Then the semen is diluted with a sterile solution, placed in thin tubes known as straws, and frozen in liquid nitrogen. Six to eight specimens are collected, with at least two days elapsing between ejaculations, which can be stored for five years or more and used any time for attempts at insemination.

The sperm usually survives the freezing process remarkably well, and many normal pregnancies have resulted from insemination with frozen sperm, although the procedure is not very pleasant or dignified for the woman.

A variation on this theme, useful if the freezing system fails for one reason or another, is for the man to have an ejaculation, then collect his urine immediately afterwards so that the sperm can be separated out and used for insemination. Again, not very dignified, but the sperm usually survives the ordeal, and many normal pregnancies have resulted from this process. Pregnancy has even been achieved by post-ejaculatory voiding into the vagina.

Bleeding

As we have seen in the previous chapter, there are a number of short-term side-effects after the operation, mainly related to bleeding and infection. Occasionally, bleeding is severe enough to require transfusions and a longer stay in hospital.

During a TUR operation, the surgeon cauterizes bleeding blood vessels as he goes along with the same electrical instrument used to remove the prostate tissue. This leads to a scab forming during the day or two following surgery, and usually the urine is clear of all visible bleeding by the third or fourth postoperative day. By the time the scab falls off two or three weeks later, the blood vessel will normally have healed.

Occasionally, the scab may fall off too early, resulting in renewed bleeding which is sometimes quite heavy – heavy enough to require readmission to hospital. This usually occurs because the patient has exerted himself in some way, raising his abdominal blood pressure, which is one reason why he is told to take things easy for up to six weeks after the operation even when he feels more or less back to normal.

Healing is promoted by a good through-put of dilute urine, which washes out the blood and any small pieces of scab. If a man tends to suffer from constipation, a stool-softener will usually be given to prevent him straining on the toilet.

TUR syndrome

A rare but unpleasant immediate complication of TUR surgery is a condition known as 'TUR syndrome'. This occurs immediately after the operation, and is characterized by swelling of the limbs and sometimes confusion. It is caused by absorption of the special irrigating fluid used during the operation (often glycine), which has to be non-conducting. It is treated with special diuretics and usually clears up in a day or two, although it will delay discharge from hospital. Once it has cleared up, it will not recur.

Longer-term problems

For some patients, problems persist for three months or more. One large US study found that as many as 15 per cent of men had one or more episodes of acute retention due to blood clots within three months of their prostatectomy; 20 per cent had a post-surgical infection, which lasted for two or more weeks in

7 per cent of cases. Altogether, a quarter of all patients reported a non-routine visit to their doctors for prostate-related problems, and 8 per cent were readmitted to hospital.

The US study found evidence of continuing problems on a
smaller scale after three months. From the fourth to the 12th
month after surgery, 11 per cent of men reported visits to their
doctor for prostate problems and 3 per cent were readmitted to
hospital for the same reason.

Other studies have found a mortality rate of over 4 per cent
in the three months after leaving hospital, and rates of urethral
scarring of between 4 and 16 per cent. At least 5 per cent of
men who were sexually active before the operation report
problems with having erections afterwards.

Some scientists have suggested that, despite its apparent
advantages, the TUR operation might be less successful than
open operations in some respects. An international study looking at the outcome for over 50,000 men who had undergone
prostate operations in Denmark, England and Canada found
that the men who had had a TUR seemed to have a slightly
higher risk of dying (of other causes, particularly heart
attacks) during the five years following the operation than men
who had had an open prostatectomy.

What is more, they also had a higher risk of having to
undergo a second prostate operation. At eight years after the
first operation, this risk was 12 per cent in Denmark as against
4.5 per cent for those having had open surgery, 15.5 per cent in
Canada as against 4.2, and 12 per cent in England as against
1.8.

In open surgery, it is of course easier to be sure of removing
all the prostate tissue, since this is 'enucleated' as described in
Chapter 2; this provides a reasonable explanation for the higher rate of reoperation in the TUR group. Some urologists main-
tain that, in good hands, a TUR can be just as effective in
removing tissue, and suggest that this study does not reflect
the best TUR practice, and in any case covered cases operated
on nearly 20 years ago, since when further progress in TUR
technique has been made. Others agree that a retropubic
operation removes more tissue, and believe there is a good
case for doing a retropubic rather than a TUR on a younger
man with a large gland.

The higher mortality finding is more of a puzzle, and the
authors admit that it 'may prove to be a consequence of

unmeasured characteristics of patients'. Another possible explanation may lie in the nature of the irrigating fluid used in TUR which is known to be sometimes absorbed into the blood stream during the operation, causing 'TUR syndrome'.

If so, this may prove to be less of a problem in the future, as other less toxic irrigating fluids are now commonly used and the modern resectoscope requires a lower pressure of irrigating fluid to be maintained, which means that less fluid enters the bloodstream. Certainly, TUR syndrome is less common today than it was 15 years ago.

Incontinence

The most unpleasant complication of prostatectomy, and the one dreaded almost as much as impotence, is incontinence. True incontinence, where the man is unable to hold his water at all and has to wear an incontinence device, is very uncommon after TUR; but some degree of incontinence – occasioned by stress, running or coughing, for instance – is not unusual, especially in the months following surgery. In the US study quoted above, as many as 20 per cent of men reported a problem with dripping at one time or another during the year following the operation, and for 4 per cent of these it was a continuous problem.

True incontinence usually only occurs when the external sphincter or the muscles surrounding the prostatic capsule are damaged during surgery. This should not happen in the hands of a skilled surgeon, but some surgeons are inevitably less experienced than others, and their inexperience may sometimes be compounded by heavy bleeding which prevents them seeing exactly what tissue they are removing.

Slight incontinence problems often right themselves with time, and can be helped by drug therapy. Drugs like ephedrine or pseudoephedrine act on the muscles surrounding the prostate capsule, making it contract and reducing the size of the prostatic urethra, which of course is considerably widened by surgery although it does shrink after a time. Other drugs can relax the bladder and prevent it from contracting so readily.

In the case of a damaged sphincter, repair surgery is often possible. Another possibility, developed primarily for total incontinence arising from other causes, is an artificial sphincter, implanted surgically to surround the urethra next to the true sphincter. The sphincter is a circular cuff connected to a pump mechanism buried in the upper part of the scrotum and a reservoir placed under the muscles of the lower abdomen. The cuff is kept inflated; when the man wishes to urinate, he presses a button on the pump in his scrotum which allows fluid to go from the cuff into the reservoir, deflating the cuff and allowing urine to flow. Thirty seconds after the button is pressed, the cuff automatically reflates.

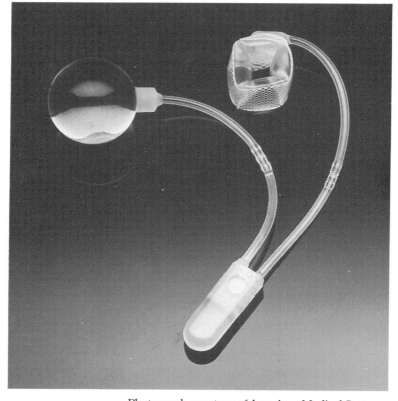

Photograph courtesy of American Medical Systems
Fig. 4.1: artificial sphincter

There are a number of other solutions available for men who are less seriously affected: incontinence pads, clamps, pouches and bags. Some degree of incontinence is quite common in the elderly, and the appliances that have been developed make life a lot easier and less embarrassing.

Stricture

'Stricture' means narrowing of the urethra by scarring caused by damage or infection. Confronted by evidence of urinary obstruction, one of the first things the urologist must be sure is that it is not caused by stricture, which can be easily remedied but can produce symptoms similar to prostate obstruction.

Unfortunately, one of the hazards of transurethral surgery is damage to the urethra, which can cause a stricture with its own obstructive symptoms, perhaps as bad or even worse than that previously caused by his prostate. It is caused by the urethral channel being too narrow for the resectoscope used for the operation.

What usually happens nowadays is that the surgeon measures the bore of the urethra before beginning surgery; if it proves too narrow for the instrument, he then makes a little slit to widen it at the narrowest part (*urethrotomy*). The operation then goes ahead without causing further damage.

One estimate is that some 10 to 15 per cent of men having a TUR suffer some damage to the urethra as a result of the operation. This proportion is reduced considerably where surgeons carry out a preliminary gauging of the urethra. Even when it does occur, it may not necessarily create problems: the narrowing may be too insignificant to create outflow obstruction.

When strictures do occur, they can often be stretched periodically (*dilatation*), which is a quick and fairly painless procedure. Occasionally, minor surgery is needed, either to allow the urethra to heal around a catheter, or to repair the stricture with plastic surgery.

Strictures do also occasionally occur after the open retropubic operation at the point where the urethra is divided to remove the enlarged tissue, if the cut is not done cleanly and sharply.

Acute retention

It is not unusual for acute retention of urine to occur not long after the operation. This is disconcerting, especially if it happens after you have gone home from hospital, since acute retention is one of the conditions which the operation is supposed to cure, and may indeed have been the immediate cause of the decision to operate.

Although unpleasant, acute retention after the operation is not as serious as it seems. It is often caused, if within a few days of the operation, by a blood clot obstructing the bladder exit. Catheterization and a bladder wash-out quickly put things right. It can also be caused by an infection flaring up, and this can be cleared up by antibiotics. It is rare for acute retention to recur once the prostate area has healed after the operation.

Epididymitis

This is an unpleasant but now fairly rare complication of prostate surgery, which occasionally occurs two to six weeks following surgery. The symptoms are pain and enlargement of one or both testicles, caused by infection and inflammation of the epididymis, the cord-like structure alongside the testicles where the sperm are stored and mature.

It happens because an infection from the operation site travels up the vas (sperm canal) to the testicle. It usually only occurs if the patient has a urinary tract infection at the time of the operation. It is treated with antibiotics and painkillers, which reduces the acute discomfort in a week or two, but the swelling can take much longer to go down.

Bladder neck contracture

This is a rare but troublesome complication of TUR surgery, in which the bladder neck is injured during the operation and contracts when it heals and scars. This tends to occur only during removal of small enlargements of the prostate, which in any case are less likely to be surgically treated today.

The small bladder opening that results is often worse than that caused by prostatic enlargement (sometimes as small as a pinhead), and must be enlarged by further surgery. The surgery may need to be repeated in the future, because the narrowing tends to recur.

Sexual problems

There is no convincing reason why a prostate operation should leave a man with sexual problems. It is known that all surgery on elderly men – even tooth extractions – can occasionally precipitate impotence, or at least lack of interest in sex.

Prostate surgery does of course involve the male sexual area, but nothing occurs in a TUR prostate operation which should affect sexuality in any way – except retrograde ejaculation. There is absolutely nothing in a TUR procedure which should alter libido or prevent a man from getting or maintaining an erection, since a TUR is limited to removing tissue within the prostate capsule and cannot damage the nerve bundles controlling erection which are outside the prostate capsule. Yet it does seem occasionally to happen. Why?

One obvious explanation is that some men may use the operation as a pretext for avoiding sex which they no longer really enjoy. Sometimes, especially if a man is not in very strong health generally, a prostate operation, which is a major operation and one which requires a longish convalescence even for younger men, may prove the last straw for sexual activity: he may just not feel up to it afterwards.

But generally, a man who has a loving sexual relationship before his operation, will not have any problems after it. Indeed, his sex life may improve, since he will feel better with a bladder that empties properly and kidneys that are no longer under stress.

Potency aids

For the sake of completeness, descriptions are given here of some of the modern aids and prostheses which are now available to men who have lost their potency, for whatever reason, but wish to continue with sexual intercourse. It is important to realize that most men who have lost their erective function still retain the ability to have orgasm and ejaculate (providing they don't have retrograde ejaculation, of course).

Often impotence is not truly organic impotence (when erection is functionally impossible) but is psychologically generated. In the case of psychogenic impotence, erections continue

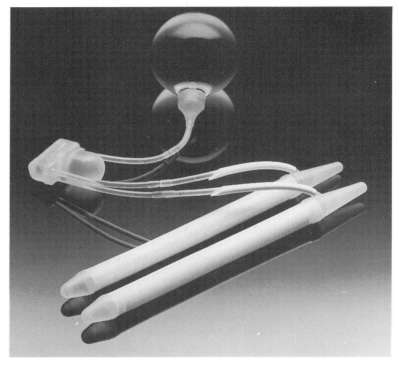

Photograph courtesy of American Medical Systems
Fig. 4.2: inflatable penile prosthesis

to occur when the man is asleep, but he is unable to achieve an erection when he is awake.

A drug which is widely used to help men with erective problems, especially in the United States (although it does not yet have Food and Drug Administration approval), is *papaverine*, a drug derived, like morphine, from the oriental poppy. When injected into the shaft of the penis, it causes an increase in the blood supply which usually results in an erection.

The injections are first done by the urologist, then the man learns to do them himself. He can use it up to 10 or 12 times a month, and most men find that it results in excellent erections, which last for one or two hours. In fact, what papaverine induces is priapism, not a true erection, and the glans of the penis does not become erect, only the shaft. But it has proved a boon to many men and their wives, and does not seem to cause any side-effects. There is however a possible complication in men who are particularly sensitive to the drug: erections in this case may last for more than an hour or two, and the urologist must be on the lookout for this when first using the drug, because erections lasting more than four or five hours can cause permanent damage to the penis.

Some men prefer to have a *prosthetic implant*. One type of penile implant is a semi-rigid plastic device, which makes the penis always rigid, but can be bent downward (normally) or upward (for intercourse). This is a simple device, fitted by straightforward surgery into the spongy part of the penis, which has no working parts to go wrong.

A more sophisticated implant is the inflatable variety, which allows for an increase in girth as well as rigidity of the penis. The most frequently used device has a pump, placed in the scrotum, which transfers fluid from a reservoir placed in the abdomen to paired cylinders implanted in the penis. The pump is activated by squeezing, and when the erection is no longer desired, a release valve on the pump allows the return of fluid from the cylinders to the reservoir (see Figs. 4.2 and 4.3).

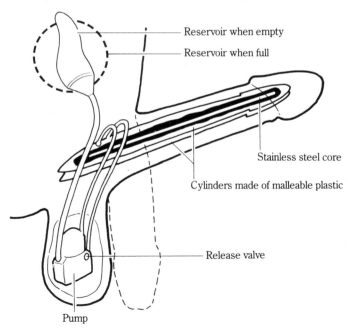

Fig. 4.3: inflatable penile prosthesis in situ

Another device which dispenses with surgery is a rigid plastic phallus-shaped cover for the penis, which is lubricated and placed snugly over the penis. The slack penis is fitted into the device through a vacuum being formed through sucking on a silicon tube, the vacuum then maintained by a cover on the tube. The front under-side of the device is thinner, permitting much the same sort of sensitivity as a condom. Manufactured in West Germany under the trade mark 'Correctaid', the device has to be made to measure.

Reoperation

Most men blithely assume that, once done, a prostate operation will last for life. Fortunately this is true for the vast majority, but in some men the prostate tissue does grow back sufficiently in their lifetime to necessitate further surgery. This happened to Ronald Reagan, who had a second prostate operation under an epidural while he was in his first term as President: with Nancy on his arm, he was shown on television disappearing into Washington's Bethesda Naval Hospital with the cheery quip, 'We've been here before!'

What happens is that after the removal of the prostate tissue in the operation, the prostate capsule tends to shrink and effectively become part of the urethra. When the adenoma (benign tumorous tissue) grows again, as it usually does, it does not need to grow so far as before to obstruct the urine flow. Occasionally, it grows back very quickly. Mr Mike G. writes: 'Twice over the years I've been in hospital having my prostate "reamed out" (my words), the last time only a year ago. Today it's as bad as ever again. It seems to me a very primitive way of getting water to flow again.' As we have seen above, up to 15 per cent of men who have had a TUR prostatectomy may need to have a second operation within eight years; the proportion is higher for men, like Ronald Reagan, who have their first operation before they are 60.

Quality of life

The proportion of men in a given age group who undergo a prostate operation varies considerably from country to country, and even from region to region within particular countries. This cannot reflect a different incidence of prostate enlargement, and is most probably due to the different views taken by different groups of urologists as to exactly what symptoms and circumstances would lead to the need for surgery.

In the United States, for instance, three times the proportion of men over 60 receive a prostatectomy than receive it in Britain. Several factors can help explain this:

- An American urologist gets a fee of, say, $1,000 for each prostatectomy, so he is motivated to do as many as possible. A British urologist will do most of his surgery under the National Health Service, so is not financially motivated to operate; he may have a huge waiting list and will probably only do a prostatectomy on patients with bad symptoms. A similar process probably accounts for the higher rate of caesareans and hysterectomies carried out in the United States.
- British hospitals are overburdened and have long waiting lists for non-urgent surgery. A few hospitals have given up doing routine prostate operations altogether, so their patients go untreated or swell waiting lists elsewhere.
- There is professional uncertainty about how to treat prostate problems, and about which symptoms justify surgery. This is likely to increase in the future as more non-surgical treatments become available (see Chapter 5).

A study carried out in the US state of Maine on the effects of prostatectomy in improving symptoms and patients' quality of life found that different men reacted differently to the same symptoms. Some worried more about their health in general, some felt more limited by their prostate symptoms in their day-to-day activities, and a substantial number of severely symptomatic patients were not very concerned about their condition. Generally, the study found that prostatectomy proved effective in reducing symptoms for most patients, with 78 per cent of those followed up reporting only mild symptoms a year after surgery. But for a minority, symptoms remained the same or got worse; and 20 per cent of those who were mildly symptomatic before the operation reported moderate or severe symptoms at the end of the year.

The conclusion of the study is that TUR patients with severe symptoms before the operation, perhaps not surprisingly, show the greatest improvement. But for those operated on for moderate or mild symptoms, there was no statistical improvement of quality of life – and some had negative effects. Even men who have had an episode of acute retention, considered by many urologists, especially in Britain, to be an absolute indication for prostatectomy, may do just as well after a period of catheter drainage as after an operation, according to the Maine study.

It seems to be important therefore for both urologists and patients not to expect too much from prostate surgery. True, for many cases there are clear-cut medical reasons for surgery – chronic retention of large volumes of urine and any impairment of kidney function – and these will almost always benefit, both from the health and quality of life point of view.

For men with less clear-cut symptoms, this chapter should certainly not be read as an argument against them seeking medical advice. It is always best to err on the side of caution in consulting the doctor, who may simply be able to reassure that nothing is seriously amiss. But, with several types of non-surgical treatment already being tried out (see Chapter 5), there may be a case for arguing with your consultant against immediate surgery if he agrees that this is not essential.

Case history 4.1

Mr Vincent R. first had some of the classic symptoms of prostate trouble in his late 70s: 'having to get up perhaps three or four times during the night, passing water in the course of a social evening, and then a few minutes later having to repeat the process'.

'Eventually' he sought medical advice and after a delay of only a few weeks was admitted for a prostatectomy. He was then 82. The operation at that time seemed to have been successful, but within a few months problems arose.

'I had a sort of dribbling, for want of a better word, which was occasional, not continuous. Then perhaps during the course of a social evening, my urine wanted out, and out it came, and all my will power could not prevent this. This happens a few times a week.

'I have gradually learnt to live with these symptoms by watching my fluid intake. For instance, when I go to church on a Sunday morning, I have only one cup of tea, and this seems to be effective.

'I have not had a holiday for years, nor have I been to a cinema or theatre, and I always try to have friends visit me rather than go to them. I am now 83, and could probably go back to St Thomas's for some sort of repair job, but I just can't be bothered.'

Case history 4.2

Mr Paul L. had a transurethral prostate operation when he was in his early 70s, which seemed to go well. The only semi-serious after-effects were excessive tiredness and bouts of depression, but this had to do (I was told) with the anaesthetic; it took me the best part of three months to get back to normal.

'For a few years I felt fine and vastly relieved by not having to get up in the night to pee and not having to consider my bladder when travelling or going to a theatre, etc. I also considered myself lucky as the sexual apparatus remained completely unimpaired by the operation.

'But after a few years I began to wake up in the middle of the night with the urge to empty my bladder. I was told by my GP that "one pee a night" was perfectly normal and nothing to worry about. However, after a while one became two, and later three – sometimes four.

'I am now 79 years old. The state of my heart and of my bronchia leaves much to be desired. I dread the possibility of any kind of operation. My present GP thinks I should only see the urologists when my prostate gives serious trouble. I decided that "serious" means either acute retention or "dribbling", but that waking up every two hours is not. I no longer drive long distances. So if I am lucky, either my heart or my respiratory system will give out before my prostate.'

Case history 4.3

Mr James C. suffered from prostatitis and benign enlargement. At the age of 60 he noticed some blood in his ejaculate (not an unusual occurrence with prostatitis) and was told to enter hospital for a prostate operation. 'Having gone through all the pre-op tests, I was told I could not have the operation without an AIDS test as I am a homosexual. The senior sexually transmitted disease consultant could not have been more kind, and did the test there and then.

'After the operation I did have a very trying time as my catheter kept blocking up and I was frequently in extreme discomfort and indeed pain. As a result I developed a bladder infection which delayed my discharge. My recovery at home was rather slow and just as I felt the worst was over I had a bladder retention and had to be rushed into hospital at midnight because I could not urinate. After a long and painful wait I was fitted with a catheter, but during the next two days I had exactly the same problem as before – frequent blocking of the catheter and another infection. Despite this, no one from the consultant's team visited me.

'Eventually it all cleared up. On the credit side, despite the consultant's warning, I *can* still ejaculate outwardly, albeit a reduced quantity and with a delayed reaction. On the debit side, I seem to have frequent bouts of tenderness and irritation in the urethra, a certain numbness of the penis at times, and a general feeling that all is not as it should be.'

CHAPTER 5

Non-surgical treatment for benign enlargement: progress and prospects

For centuries, doctors have tried to find non-surgical treatment for prostate enlargement. The common nature of the complaint, and the dangers and drawbacks of surgery provided ample incentives for them to do so. But until quite recently their attempts had met with almost complete failure.

In the past ten years or so, several promising lines of research have opened up, and although it is safe to say that none is likely to provide a 'cure' for all cases of urinary obstruction caused by benign enlargement, the prospects for at least a proportion of patients to be able to have effective non-surgical treatment within the next five or ten years are genuinely good.

In fact, one leading London urologist believes that we are now at a turning point in the treatment of benign enlargement. As with hypertension (high blood pressure) 15 years ago, we are on the brink of moving from one basic treatment to a range of therapies, with some treatments more effective for some forms of the complaint. Some of the new treatments also hold out promise for certain sufferers of prostatitis and prostate cancer, and these will also be mentioned in this chapter.

Leaving aside alternative or complementary medical treatments, such as acupuncture and homoeopathy, which will be dealt with in Chapter 7, these new treatments fall into three basic categories:

- *pills*
- *mechanical methods* of improving flow through the prostate without removing tissue
- *hyperthermia* or heat treatment.

Few people would undergo a major operation if they could achieve a similar effect by taking a pill every day or undergoing a course of outpatient treatment every few years. Yet even the most enthusiastic proponent of any of these non-surgical methods would hesitate to claim better than a 50 per cent success rate – and then the effect may not be permanent (although as we have seen in Chapter 4, the effect of the prostate operation may not always be permanent either).

But there are certain groups of men who are particularly well suited for non-surgical treatment, even if the effect is inferior to that likely to be achieved by a prostatectomy. They are:

- Men who are unsuitable for major surgery because of heart, circulatory or lung problems, and are unsuitable or too weak for the transurethral operation to be done under spinal anaesthesia;
- Men with arthritis of the hips and knees making it difficult to place them in the correct position for transurethral surgery;
- Men who wish to avoid the operation and the retrograde ejaculation it normally brings because they wish (or may wish) to have (more) children.

To these three main groups could be added those men who, for no medically convincing reason, wish to avoid surgery, or simply preserve their power to ejaculate. Together, these categories add up to a substantial number of men, which would be hugely swollen if everybody was told that they might be able to avoid surgery by trying one of these other treatments.

Examples of men unsuitable for surgery are Mr Bill S. of County Durham, who writes: 'I am catheterized, and the consultant and her colleagues have advised against an operation as I am suffering from heart disease. Needless to say, I suffer excruciating pain many, many times a day.' And M. Jacques D. of Paris, aged 61, also catheterized, who cannot be operated on as he has just had a second heart attack, and has weak lungs. Mr David H. of London on the other hand is a fit 51-year-old who is threatened with prostatectomy because of one episode of acute retention. he and his younger wife want to have another baby, but retrograde ejaculation would put paid to that. 'All the consultant can suggest is banking semen, followed by a "conservative" prostatectomy, in the hope that ejaculation is preserved. He says there's no other option.'

Non-surgical therapies over the years have been many and various. Hot water irrigation into the rectum or through the urethra was supposed to relieve the symptoms. Electrical massage and galvanic stimulation were used in the last century, and quartz light therapy in the 1920s. Shortwave diathermy, X-ray irradiation, the introduction of radium needles into the prostate through the rectum or urethra, were all tried with little apparent success.

Other urologists tried injecting the prostate with 'biological agents', some containing fresh prostate extract or testicular extract. Another approach was to attempt 'sclerosis' of the gland by injecting it with a mixture of phenol or carbolic acid, glacial acetic acid and glycerin. Some patients were relieved, but others developed abscesses and a few died. Pills were also tried – some with bizarre ingredients: French doctors in the last century tried a mixture of strychnine, centaury (a plant extract) and gentian powder, and prescription of ergot, lithium carbonate and witchhazel. Sodium iodide was fashionable for a time.

It has clearly not been for the want of trying that non-surgical treatments have proved so elusive to the medical profession. It seems that some patients did definitely benefit from some of these therapies, but no treatment proved able to provide safe, consistent and long-lasting relief. But today we do seem to be a bit closer to this objective, although the ideal treatment, for most patients, still seems as elusive as ever. Let us first look at recent pharmaceutical approaches.

Pills

Some early attempts to treat BPH centred on the fact that the condition is androgen-dependent: men castrated before the age of 40 do not develop prostatic enlargement. Members of an obscure religious sect in Russia who were castrated at the age of 35 never developed benign enlargement. Castration was tried in the 1890s as a means of treatment, and improvement in symptoms and some prostate shrinkage was reported; but the procedure did not prove popular, and when safe prostate operations were developed, interest in this approach waned.

But in the last decade, research into the action of luteinizing-hormone-releasing hormone (LHRH), which plays a key role in reproduction in both men and women, has led to renewed interest in the effects of androgens on the prostate. This is because LHRH effectively controls the level of androgens in the blood in men. (It also controls the process of ovulation in women, and this function is the basis for a promising line of contraceptive research.) In 1987, a team at Johns Hopkins University School of Medicine found that implanting a slow-release capsule of a drug called *nafarelin acetate* under the skin caused the enlarged prostate to shrink by 24 per cent and resulted in a 30 per cent improvement in urine flow rates. Nafarelin acetate is an LHRH agonist – a drug which mimics the action of LHRH.

Other researchers have claimed even better results with different LHRH agonists. But when the treatment stops, the prostate returns to its pre-treatment size within six months, and – more seriously – patients experience a loss of libido and often impotence during treatment. This is not surprising, since this is an androgen-deprivation treatment – a temporary chemical castration.

So although it works to some extent, androgen deprivation has limited application in the treatment of benign enlargement. Another line of drug research is based on the discovery, in the 1940s, that enlarged prostates contained high levels of cholesterol. Over the last 15 years, various cholesterol-lowering drugs have been given to prostate patients. The most widely-used substance is called *Candicidin*, and this is still prescribed in France and some other European countries, but the results have not been promising enough to persuade British and American urologists that it is much use.

Most attention during the 1980s focused on attempting to influence the muscular elements of the prostate and bladder neck through so-called *alpha-blockers*. Around 40 per cent of the volume of the prostate consists of muscular fibre or stroma, and in some of the smaller, 'fibrous' prostates causing obstruction, the proportion is higher. These muscles are influenced by the amounts of certain adrenalin by-products circulating in the blood, and alpha-blockers inhibit the take-up of these substances.

The first drug of this nature to be tried was *phenoxybenzamine* (PXB). This worked quite well in terms of reducing symptoms, but because it is a non-specific alpha-blocker, it had unwanted side-effects such as nasal stuffiness and low blood pressure in 30 per cent of patients. These, and reports that PXB caused cancer in rats, were enough to have the drug withdrawn for the treatment of benign enlargement.

A few years later, a selective alpha-blocker, *Prazosin*, was launched, and has proved much more suitable. It produces better results than PXB and virtually none of the side-effects. A study of patients with prostatic obstruction, carried out by the Middlesex Hospital, London, in 1986, showed that prazosin taken over four weeks greatly improved the urinary flow rate (by an average of 60 per cent), and also reduced the patients' frequency by day and night. In most of the men there was also an increase in bladder capacity. No one in the study complained of impotence or other sexual problems, there was no incidence of low blood pressure. However, retrograde ejaculation is likely to occur with such drugs, something that urologists do not always consider worth mentioning.

Prazosin is now generally available and can be prescribed by general practitioners. It is not a cure, since its use does not seem to help with the reduction of residual urine volumes. And it does not produce such a marked improvement in urine flow rates as prostatectomy does; this is because Prazosin works by relaxing muscles in the bladder neck and the prostate, but obviously does not reduce the bulk of the enlarged gland, which is probably the main cause of the increased resistance to urinary flow in most patients.

But it certainly has a role in the treatment of men with moderate obstruction (who may not always require surgery), and of those who are on the waiting list for surgery or who are unfit for the operation. Other similar formulations are also available, such as *Doxasosin* (a once-a-day pill), *Terazosin* and *Indoramin*.

Another alpha-blocker, *Alfuzosine*, is slightly different, as it is a competitive blocker of the contractions of the bladder and upper urethra. It is especially effective when there is pain on urination (dysuria).

Undoubtedly the most exciting line of research in recent

years has been into the function of a number of substances which actually have the effect of shrinking the enlarged prostate. These work on the principle that the adenoma, or benign tumorous growth of the prostate, is dependent not directly on the male hormone testosterone, but on a metabolite of the hormone called dihydro-testosterone (DHT). Any substance which inhibits the action of the steroid which converts testosterone into DHT could have the effect of reducing the size of the enlarged prostate.

Two major drug companies are spending hundreds of millions of dollars in the development of pills to do just this. Trials are in progress now, and the first pill is expected to be on the market by 1994. Both these pills contain substances which inhibit the action of steroid 5-alpha reductase, the enzyme which converts testosterone into DHT. As this book goes to press, Merck Sharp & Dohme, the world's largest pharmaceutical company, has completed Phase III trials in several countries – that is, large-scale trials on volunteer patients. The results are not yet published, but it is clear that a very small dose (5 mg) twice a day of the new drug, called Proscar (or by its generic name, finasteride), has a dramatic effect in about 40 per cent of men with benign enlargement, actually shrinking the prostate by about 30 per cent, and improving urinary flow rates and other symptoms to near normal parameters.

The majority of the men taking the pill in the trials did show substantial improvement, but some did not. Since this drug works by shrinking the adenoma (tumorous enlargement), those men whose prostates are obstructive mainly because of excess muscular fibre are unlikely to be helped very much: they are probably better treated with a selective alpha-blocker like Prazosin which acts on muscle tissue (see above).

Another large US drug company, Smith Kline & French (now merged with the British Beecham group), has developed a similar, but not identical, 5-alpha reductase inhibitor. They are a year or two behind Merck, but by the time this book is published Phase III (large-scale human volunteer) trials will be in progress. Smith Kline believe that their inhibitor may prove to have an advantage in some patients over finasteride. This is because finasteride is one of a group of 'competitive' inhibitors whose action can theoretically be reduced by the presence of high concentrations of testosterone. Since the inhibition of DHT production results in the availability of extra quantities of testosterone, this is a potential problem. The Smith Kline drug is an 'uncompetitive' inhibitor whose action is unaffected by high levels of testosterone.

Whether or not one drug proves superior to the other, it is clearly healthy for two companies to be pursuing the same goal, and likely to result in cheaper treatment costs eventually. Possible long-term problems may emerge in the use of these drugs because of the quantities of unconverted testosterone, which tend to collect in the prostate, resulting in perhaps a 700 per cent increase in testosterone in the prostate. However, none has been detected so far.

The background to the research carried out by these two drug companies is interesting. The identification of dihydro-testosterone (DHT), rather than testosterone itself, as a causative factor in the development and progression of benign prostate enlargement resulted from the study of a rare human genetic deficiency. Some males are born genetically deficient in steroid 5-alpha reductase, the enzyme which converts testosterone to DHT. It was the study of this genetic deficiency which suggested a strategy for suppressing 5-alpha reductase by pharmacological means.

Males with steroid 5-alpha reductase deficiency are born with ambiguous external genitalia and are commonly raised as girls. At puberty, there is a striking change with the development of a functional male penis, enlarged scrotum, increase in muscle mass and the male voice change. This genetic deficiency is relatively common in the Dominican Republic, where it was identified in the 1970s. Affected males are referred to locally as *guevedoces* ('penis at age 12'). In adolescence and adulthood, these individuals only develop a tiny prostate, their hairline does not recede, and they never get acne. This deficiency enabled researchers to identify which androgen is responsible for which effect in male development:

Testosterone-induced	**DHT-induced**
Male sex drive	Increased facial and body hair
Muscle mass increase	Acne
Penis enlargement	Male baldness
Scrotum enlargement	Prostate enlargement
Vocal cord enlargement	
Sperm production	

DHT depletion, through inhibition of its conversion from testosterone, can be therefore expected to have positive therapeutic effects without having adverse consequences on the masculine characteristics produced by testosterone. It also seems likely that these inhibitors will have other therapeutic uses. Animal experiments have suggested that an inhibitor can help prevent the spread of prostate cancer, can prevent baldness when applied to the scalp of a male monkey, and may be able to treat acne and hirsutism (excessive hairiness) in women and girls.

There seems to be no evidence to suggest that acne, excessive body hair, or premature baldness are directly linked with prostate enlargement. (In other words, a man who goes bald early is not necessarily going to suffer from early prostate problems.) But it is possible that these new pills, as well as in many cases reducing the size of enlarged prostates and the symptoms they cause, may also at the same time promote new hair growth on the scalp or at least prevent further baldness occurring.

Unlike a prostatectomy (although this operation sometimes has to be repeated), 5-alpha reductase inhibitors are not a one-off treatment: it seems likely that affected men will have to continue to take the pills for the rest of their lives, because once you stop taking the drug, the prostate enlarges to its previous size within a week or so. Unappealing as this prospect may be, the evidence so far is that side-effects are absent, since the pill seems to act solely on prostate tissue. It is worth recalling that patients with other conditions, such as high blood pressure, heart conditions and diabetes, have for many years been taking daily medication, often *with* side-effects, and the quality of their lives has been improved thereby.

These pills may well prove to provide an effective alternative to surgery in many cases of prostatic obstruction. But they do not seem to work in all cases. And other lines of treatment are continuing to be tried out. Let us first look at treatments which use mechanical means of dealing with the obstruction. The main method is the fitting of a stent, a metal spring or perforated tube to hold the urethra open as it passes through the prostate.

Stents

The idea that some kind of tube could be inserted in the prostatic urethra so that it is no longer 'squashed' by the pressure of the enlarged prostate, is a common-sense one.

But researchers have been hindered by two main problems which arise when a foreign body is inserted into the urethra or bladder. These problems are infection and encrustation.

Urine is an ideal medium for bacteria to grow in, and anything inserted, whether a suture, an instrument or whatever, is likely to generate infection. Urine is also a solution of salts, more saturated at some times than at others, and these salts are very liable to crystallize out onto any foreign body; this in fact is how bladder stones are formed, calcium deposits building up in the constant presence of urine not completely emptied from the bladder around a tiny piece of tissue or impurity.

Urologists (and cardiologists) have used tubes or metallic coils called 'stents' to hold open the constricted bodily passage. They have been used in urology to overcome strictures – narrowing of the urethra caused by injury or disease. But the problem of encrustation has meant that they have had to be changed regularly, so they must be designed in such a way that they can be easily removed.

Two types of stents are currently under trial, and results are encouraging, although few urologists would suggest that they are likely to be used in the future as the standard alternative to conventional prostatectomy.

The first is the *Fabian Urospiral* (see Fig. 5.1), developed in West Germany by a urologist called Fabian. A similar device is called Prostakath. This is a flexible spiral which keeps the prostatic urethra open. These stents are now plated with silver or gold to discourage encrustation, but they do eventually have to be changed. However, both placing and removal is quick and easy, taking no more than 10 minutes under local anaesthesia.

Researchers believe that the procedure is indicated in five

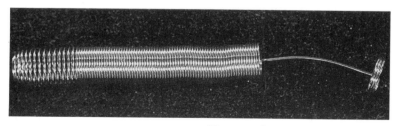

Photograph courtesy of Porgès SA

Fig. 5.1: urospiral stent

groups of patient: those who are medically unfit for surgery; those who have cancer and a short life expectancy; those patients in whom the prostate operation may well not improve their condition (patients with dementia, Parkinson's disease, or severe diabetes, for instance); patients who require catheterization for a few weeks before operations; and younger patients who have urinary obstruction but are keen to avoid retrograde ejaculation.

This particular type of stent does not hold open the bladder neck, so does not usually induce retrograde ejaculation. Its disadvantage is that it is too narrow to permit catheterization or endoscopic examination of the bladder, but this is compensated for by the ease with which it can be removed or moved.

The second type of stent currently under trial overcomes the problem of encrustation and is intended to be permanent. It is also wider than the Fabian stent, allowing endoscopic inspection of the bladder, but its use causes retrograde ejaculation because it prevents the closure of the bladder neck sphincter. Researchers are hopeful that this disadvantage can be overcome. Called the *Wallstent*, the device is made from woven fine super alloy wire. It forms a coil which is self-expanding when released from a small-diameter delivery catheter. The great advantage of this stent is that the wire it is made of is so fine that the epithelium (or skin) of the urethra actually grows over it (see Fig. 5.2).

The Wallstent has proved particularly successful in the treatment of urethral strictures. Patients with this narrowing of the urethra (which ironically sometimes results from damage sustained during transurethral prostatectomy) often have to return to their consultants again and again for stretching (dilation) or surgical widening (urethrotomy) of the part of their urethra affected, which, untreated, can cause the same symptoms and urological problems as prostate enlargement. In some cases, the stricture prevents the man ejaculating properly.

Whether for treating a stricture or prostate enlargement, the stent is inserted under local anaesthetic and guided to exactly the right position under direct vision. The results are immediate and dramatic. Within three or four months, the epithelium starts to grow over the mesh, and within six months it is completely covered. There is no scarring, the coil cannot collapse, and there seems to be no reason why it cannot

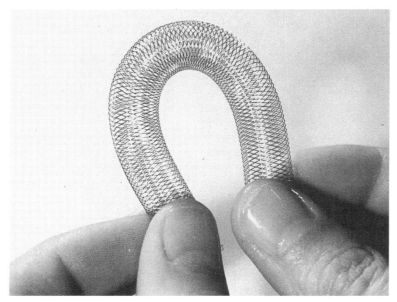

Photograph courtesy of Medinvent SA

Fig. 5.2: Wallstent

remain in position for a lifetime, like pins used to mend broken limbs or artificial hip joints.

It is possible to remove the Wallstent if it proves to have been wrongly positioned, or if it causes unexpected problems, preferably before the epithelium begins to form over it (around six to eight weeks). Another recent innovation is a titanium balloon-expandable stent.

Balloon dilatation

A rather similar idea for non-surgical relief of the obstruction caused by a swollen prostate is balloon dilatation, a procedure now quite common in the United States. For this, a special catheter containing an inflatable balloon section is inserted under local anaesthetic, the balloon is blown up, stretching the prostatic urethra to about 3–3.5 cm (1–1½") diameter, and then withdrawn.

The stretching of the prostate capsule and compacting of the prostate tissue results in a widening of the urethra and a

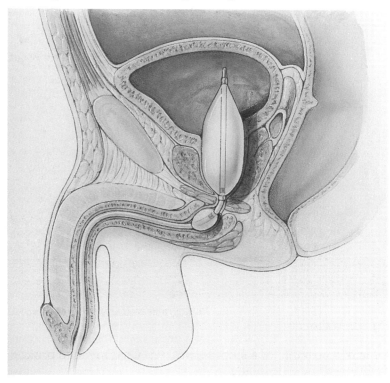

Fig. 5.3: balloon dilatation

much improved urine flow. The effect is not permanent, and may have to be repeated six months later. But the procedure is quick and can be done without anaesthetic, and is apparently harmless, so it could in theory be repeated as often as is necessary. There is some bleeding and pain, however, and urologists who do dilatation on an outpatient basis (quite common in America) do so with the patient under sedation.

Like many ideas for treating prostatic obstruction, balloon dilatation is not new, having been first tried out as early as 1812. It is reasonable to conclude that, if it was a really effective treatment, it would by now be practised more widely than it is.

In the absence of considerable improvement to these procedures, both stents and balloon dilatation seem likely to be increasingly reserved for particular classes of patient mentioned above for whom surgery is unsuitable.

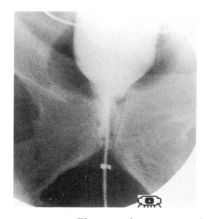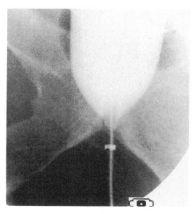

Photographs courtesy of Graham Watson/Institute of Urology
Fig. 5.4: X-rays showing balloon partially and completely inflated

Hyperthermia

Let us finally look at a new form of treatment developed in
Israel in the early 1980s and now attracting considerable interest in other countries: hyperthermia, or heating of the prostate.

The treatment, pioneered by Professor Ciro Servadio and
Dr Zvi Leib of the Beilinson Medical Centre, Petah Tiqva,
Israel, is done on an outpatient basis, and has no known side-
effects. It consists of the application of heat to the prostate
from a tiny microwave generator placed in the rectum. The
interior of the prostate is heated to around 43°C, while the generator is cooled by circulating water to prevent the bowel wall
from becoming hot. The temperature is very accurately controlled by a thermocouple placed in a catheter in the prostatic
urethra, connected to a personal computer which directs and
monitors the whole process.

It is not the first time that hyperthermia has been tried on
the prostate. An earlier treatment, developed by another
Israeli, Professor Yerushalmi, heated the prostate from a
microwave generator in a catheter in the urethra, but this tended to damage the urethra because there was no cooling system, and the temperature was difficult to control.

The success of the treatment pioneered by Servadio and
Leib seems to derive from its safety (virtually no serious side-

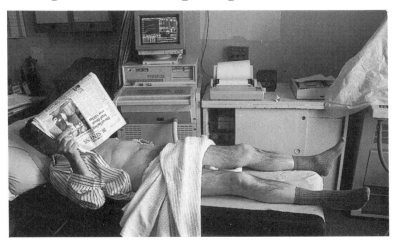

Photograph by the author

Fig. 5.5: patient undergoing hyperthermia (Primus system)

effects have been reported) and the accuracy with which the hyperthermic temperature is delivered and maintained. The equipment, called *Prostathermer*, was developed by Biodan Medical Systems of Rehovot, in conjunction with the Weizman Institute of Science. There are now over 50 Prostathermer systems in clinical use.

Normally six treatments of one hour each are given over a period of weeks, during which time the patient can lead a normal life, suffering no more than the slight discomfort of catheterization for each treatment.

Of over 1,000 men treated in Israel, only a few have received no benefit at all. The others show improvement, of varying degrees, which is known to have lasted at least two years (the normal period of follow-up). Outside Israel, trials began at the London Institute of Urology in 1989, and are also being held in France, West Germany, Spain and Italy, where as many as 14 hospitals now have the hyperthermia equipment. The Methodist Hospital of Indiana in Indianapolis is currently conducting trials as well.

First developed to help treat inoperable cancer of the prostate, the treatment has also been used to treat prostatitis (see Chapter 6). There is interest in using hyperthermia in conjunction with radiotherapy and chemotherapy in the treatment of prostate cancer (see Chapter 8).

Despite the apparent success in terms of interest and results, the treatment is still controversial. What has made many academic medical experts sceptical of the treatment is that, while it is known that heat can have a shrinking action on malignant tumours, it is not understood why hyperthermia should have an effect on a benign tumour (which is what an enlarged prostate effectively is).

In fact, the hyperthermia treatment does not always shrink a benign prostate. But it is known that symptoms, and the degree of obstruction to the urine flow caused by the prostate pressing on the urethra, are not always related to the size of the prostate, but more to the internal tonus or tension. It may be that hyperthermia has the effect of reducing this tension, an effect which can be temporarily achieved through drugs. Another possibility is that the heating changes the consistency of the prostate tissue, reducing its pressure on the urethra.

In Britain, at least, initial reactions from the always conservative urology profession were guarded, to say the least. One consultant urologist at a London teaching hospital believes the treatment is 'a waste of time'. While he thought it was 'of course right' for promising, less invasive treatments to be properly investigated, he had not been impressed by what he had read and thought that the lack of side-effects was disturbing: 'I cannot think of any effective treatment which does not have some side-effects: it suggests nothing is happening.'

Now that trials at the Institute of Urology have shown some promising results, some British consultants have changed their tune. Other urologists with direct experience of the treatment believe that the improvement recorded in many cases can only be due to some physical effect of the treatment. Professor A. Steg, in charge of the prestigious urology clinic at the Hôpital Cochin, Paris (where President de Gaulle had his prostate operation) did a study of 43 patients with severe voiding symptoms. About half his patients showed considerable objective and subjective improvement, and the study showed that those patients who had received treatment at the correct hyperthermia temperature (42.5°C or over) had done better than those who had received lower temperatures.

Professor Steg and his colleagues concluded that 'the results of this treatment are not due to a placebo effect. The effect is directly proportional to the temperature within the prostate reached during the treatment.' The team also noted a change in the consistency of the prostate after the treatment.

Some patients are unsuitable for hyperthermia treatment: those who have bladder or prostatic calculi (stones), which may reflect the microwave radiation; those whose prostate is too small, or too large; those who have stenosis or other abnormalities of the urethra; and those who have had rectal surgery (except for piles). But most patients can be treated, and they have little to lose, since the treatment does no harm, and does not involve hospitalization.

Some of the most striking authenticated cases are of men, unsuitable for operation, who have been having to wear 'indwelling' catheters – that is catheters permanently fitted, draining into a urine bag worn strapped to the thigh. Most of these men, although not cured, have been sufficiently improved for them no longer to have to wear their indwelling catheters. Other, younger, patients who wished to father additional children (difficult or impossible with the retrograde ejaculation usual after prostatectomy) have also had strikingly good results.

The improvement to the quality of life of groups of patients such as these surely justify the availability of hyperthermia equipment in major hospitals and urology clinics. The cost of the equipment is still high (from US $200,000 to $500,000), but this investment could quickly be justified by the reduced need for hospital beds and the increased productivity of men undergoing weekly outpatient treatment only. Such sums need also to be seen in the context of the cost of some drug treatments, especially those using new drugs on which there has been heavy research and development expenditure. For instance, the cost per patient of Merck's new prostate drug, Proscar, is likely to exceed US $1,000 a year and may be as high as £1,000 sterling per year. The cost of a course of hyperthermia treatment is likely to be available at well under this price, and of course does not have to be repeated every year.

In the last couple of years, there has been an upsurge of interest in the use of hyperthermia for prostate complaints. The Director of the London Institute of Urology, Mr John Wickham, believes that it is the most promising new treatment so far – more promising even than the DHT-inhibitor pills described on pages 88-90.

His optimism would seem to be borne out by the number of medical equipment manufacturers now scrambling onto the bandwagon. Companies who already produce microwave applicators for the treatment of surface tumours have launched urethral applicators of the type first developed by Yerushalmi: one, made by another Israeli manufacturer, the Thermex, is on trial at the London Institute of Urology, and another French device, the Prostatron, which raises the temperature of the prostate as high as 45°C but avoids damage to the urethra by a cooling system, is in experimental use at Charing Cross Hospital, London, and in Lyon, France. A Belgian manufacturer has developed a new type of rectal applicator which does not rely on a temperature probe in the urethra – a considerable advantage for the patient if it is proved to work accurately. This last device, the Primus, is also currently under trial at the London Institute of Urology.

Mr Wickham believes that, properly delivered, hyperthermia will be able to do what no pill can do: necrose or shrink the fibrous tissue which is such an important element of most prostatic enlargement. Already the treatment is being refined so that it can be given in fewer sessions: the Prostatron requires only one hour-long session, and the Thermex treats two patients simultaneously in a three-hour session.

Another means of delivering heat to the prostate is under trial. This is interstitial laser treatment, in which heat (and light) from a laser is transmitted via an optic fibre through a hollow needle inserted into the prostate through the perineum. This type of laser is destructive, and the effect is to cause necrosis and shrinking of the swollen tissue. Following promising trials in the United States, this procedure is now being assessed in London. Another type of laser hyperthermia being assessed at the Institute of Urology is delivered through the urethra, under light general anaesthesia.

What does seem clear from trials with different equipment is that, within reason, the higher the temperature attained within the prostate, the better the results: 43°C (as Professor Steg found) is better than 41°C, and 45°C is better than 43°C. Animal experiments have used temperatures as high as 60°C, but urologists hesitate to try such high temperatures because of the fear of ulceration. The urethral systems seem to give better results on BPH, no doubt because they heat the inner part of the prostate (where BPH occurs) more efficiently.

Hyperthermia also seems effective in treating some types of prostatitis and prostate cancer – see Chapters 6 and 8.

CHAPTER 6

Prostatitis: different types of inflammation, their causes and some treatments

Prostatitis is a catch-all expression covering various types of inflammation of the prostate. Such infections or inflammation are never as potentially serious as benign enlargement or cancer; sometimes they are easily cured, but sometimes they prove remarkably difficult to treat, and can drag on for years, quite seriously affecting a man's general health and his sex life.

Prostatitis can be acute or chronic; it can be 'bacterial' or 'non-bacterial'. Its symptoms are very variable. Sometimes a man can suffer pain and some voiding problems, without any apparent infective cause, in which case the urologist may use the term *prostatodynia*.

Chronic prostatitis can result from a dormant infection which can be identified but not eradicated; or may produce symptoms of infection without any bacteria being found. It may occasionally be caused by an allergy or by a sexually transmitted organism such as chlamydia. Sometimes it appears to be due to an infection which has spread from elsewhere in the body. It is possible that viruses or other unidentified organisms may also be responsible for prostatic inflammation; future research may clarify this. However, it may also be associated with abnormal urination causing urine to be forced into the channels of the gland.

The known causative bacteria are mainly those which always colonize the human gut and urinary tract (coliform bacteria), and can invade the prostate through infected urine or (some experts believe) by migrating through the thin layers of tissue separating the prostate from the rectum. The fungus which causes thrush in the vagina may also be occasionally implicated.

There has been some suggestion that chronic prostatitis may be brought on or made worse by jogging with a full bladder. This can cause leakage of urine into the urethra and possible reflux into the prostate.

In its various forms, prostatitis is certainly extremely common, particularly between the ages of 30 and 50, and some experts believe that as many as three-quarters of all adult males in some populations are affected by it to some degree.

Prostatitis may be present for many years without producing symptoms, then flare up for no apparent reason, and it can become a chronic complaint. In its chronic form it is not usually severe, but can become a real health nuisance, rather like chronic sinus trouble or mild arthritis, which comes and goes without any obvious cause.

Doctors sometimes dismiss prostatitis too readily, thinking that serious deterioration is unlikely and that there is little they can do. But a urodynamic investigation should always be done to rule out stones or any abnormality – including prostate cancer, which can sometimes produce symptoms similar to prostatitis.

As we have seen in Chapter 1, the prostate is a complex gland, consisting of millions of tiny sacs, lined with cells that secrete fluid, which empty into tens of thousands of tubules and ducts, and finally into the urethra through 14–18 exits. Once bacterial infection gets a hold in this dense network of sacs, tubules and tributary ducts, it is often hard to eradicate, since the body's natural defences and any medication borne by the bloodstream are unable to penetrate into every niche and crevice of the gland. The infection can remain, and flare up from time to time in the absence of treatment.

Another possible explanation for the difficulty of curing prostatitis is the presence in the outer part of the prostate of tiny calculi (stones). While large prostatic calculi are rare, small ones are quite common, and studies of calculi from men with prostatitis have shown that these are often permeated to the core with bacteria. It is easy to see how an infection can persist in the calculi within the prostate even in the presence of antibiotics, flaring up from time to time when the man is not taking antibiotics.

This is then the problem with chronic prostatitis – that the infective agent responsible for the inflammation (if it can be found) can often not be permanently eradicated. The symptoms have no correlation with any microscopical changes in the prostate. Removing the prostate tissue through prostatectomy does not usually do the trick, since the inflammation may persist in the 'capsule' left behind. It is for this reason that chronic prostatitis is known as 'the black sheep of urology': often, the urologist is powerless to bring about any lasting improvement.

Unlike benign enlargement and prostate cancer, prostatitis is not limited to middle-aged and elderly men, and quite often afflicts younger men. The inflammation usually affects the peripheral part of the prostate, not the inner part where benign enlargement occurs. It can, and often does, occur in middle-aged men in addition to benign enlargement.

Acute bacterial prostatitis

Acute bacterial prostatitis is the most dramatic form of the disease, but it is also the form that responds best to treatment. It typically strikes suddenly, with the victim developing chills, fever, pain in the lower back and perineum (area between the scrotum and the anus), and sometimes pain and difficulty in urinating.

On rectal examination, the prostate is extremely tender, and a urine test will show bacterial infection. Unlike chronic prostate infection, acute infection does respond quickly to antibiotics, probably because the intense inflammatory reaction enables the drugs to penetrate into the interior of the gland.

If the inflammation is severe enough to prevent urination altogether, the patient will have to go into hospital, where a catheter will be inserted directly into the bladder through the abdomen under local anaesthetic. With rest and antibiotics, the infection usually clears up well in a few days.

Acute bacterial prostatitis is an uncommon complaint, but when it occurs, careful follow-up is necessary to prevent the man from going on to develop chronic bacterial prostatitis, which is more common, but much more difficult to eradicate.

Chronic bacterial prostatitis

Although chronic bacterial prostatitis (CBP) sometimes develops after an earlier acute infection, it more commonly develops for no apparent reason. Its symptoms vary considerably. Some men will have pain or discomfort either in the area of the prostate, or in other areas nearby: the scrotum, testicles, penis (particularly the tip of the penis), low back, perineum (behind the scrotum), above the pubic bone, or even the inner thighs. Sometimes there is pain on ejaculation, or irritation in the 'prostate area that causes premature ejaculation, and blood is sometimes seen in the semen. Sometimes urination is affected, often not. Sometimes infection passes up the vas, causing epididymitis and swelling of a testicle. Fever and chills are unusual.

CBP is often associated with recurrent infections of the bladder or urethra, with one setting off the other. Infection of the urethra can be introduced by sexual activity, either through vaginal intercourse with a woman suffering from a urinary tract or sexually transmitted infection such as chlamydia, or through anal intercourse without a condom. This condition is known as urethritis.

Urethritis may produce similar symptoms to those listed above for CBP, and in addition often causes a slight watery discharge from the end of the penis. This is usually noticed mainly on getting up in the morning, and sometimes causes the opening of the penis to be temporarily glued shut. An infection in the urethra may migrate to the prostate and vice versa, so it is not always easy to separate the two. Any sexually transmitted disease is likely to affect the prostate and seminal vesicles.

Non-bacterial prostatitis (NBP)

Some men may have many of the symptoms of CBP described above, yet on examination no trace of any causative organism can be found. NBP is more likely to produce chronic pain in the lower abdomen, testes, base or shaft of the penis, the perineum or rectum. The medical difference between NBP and CBP is that the prostatic secretions of a patient with CBP will grow bacteria when cultured, and those of a man with NBP will contain high white cell counts but will not culture bacteria. NBP is more common than CBP. Some urologists believe there is no real difference between the two, but simply that the infection may come and go.

Prostatodynia

This expression is used to describe the condition in which some of the symptoms of prostatitis are present – mainly pain – but no bacteria and no evidence of infection such as a high white cell count can ever be found. Possible causes and treat-ments are outlined later in this chapter.

Diagnosis of prostatitis

When a man with non-acute symptoms of prostatitis comes to see his doctor, it is important to find out exactly what is causing the condition he is suffering from, so that appropriate treat-ment can be suggested. Antibiotics are only of use in treating a bacterial infection, so can help a patient with CBP, at least tem-porarily, but will do nothing at all for a man with prostatodynia.

A rectal examination does not really help in making a diagno-sis, though many urologists will do one anyway. Some urolo-gists claim that a 'boggy' prostate is a sign of bacterial infection, but modern medical thinking dismisses this on the grounds that the consistency of the prostate is variable, depending to a certain extent on the recent frequency of ejaculation, and that the rectal examination is pretty subjective anyway.

For a proper diagnosis, an examination of the prostatic fluid is necessary, and this is done by the so-called 'three-glass' pro-cess (see Fig. 6.1).

The man is asked to begin urinating into glass 1, then, with-out interrupting the stream, voids another small quantity into glass 2. Then he can urinate into the toilet, but must conscious-ly retain some urine in his bladder. Then the urologist tries to obtain a sample of prostatic fluid by massaging the prostate. For this, the patient bends over while the urologist massages his prostate through the rectum. This is sometimes painful when infection is present, and in any case is rather uncomfort-able. Sometimes some of the fluid will emerge from the penis, in which case it is collected. But more often the secretions pool in the urethra, and the patient is then asked to pass a small amount of urine into glass 3.

The contents of the three glasses are then cultured. Glass 2 will be sterile, unless a bladder infection is present. A high

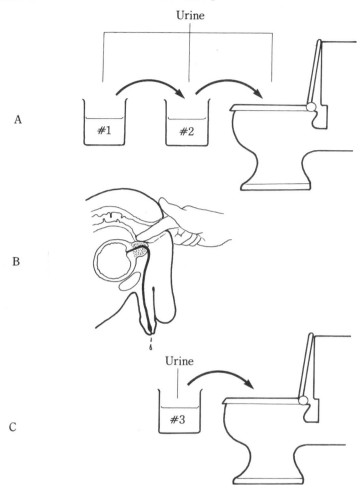

Fig. 6.1: 'three-glass' test

count of bacteria in glass 1 suggests a urethral infection. A definitive diagnosis of CBP can be made if there is at least a tenfold increase in the bacteria count in glass 3 (which contains the prostatic fluid) as compared with glass 1. If the bacteria count in glass 3 is no higher than glass 1, then non-specific urethritis is the diagnosis. If there are more bacteria in glass 2 than in glass 1, then there is a bladder infection, which must be treated with antibiotics before the test is repeated.

Often, only insignificant colonies of bacteria are found in all three glasses, although a high white cell count is found in glass 2. This means a diagnosis of NBP. If there is only a low white blood cell count in glass 2 and the patient still has symptoms, then the diagnosis is prostatodynia.

Prostatitis and fertility

There is some suspicion that some forms of prostatitis, especially CBP, may result in lower male fertility. Analysis has revealed significant changes in the physical properties and chemical constituents of the prostatic fluid of men with bacterial prostatitis.

When infection or inflammation of the prostate are present, the fluid becomes more alkaline, there is a significant reduction in the levels of zinc and prostatic antibacterial factor (PAF), and the concentrations of citric acid, an enzyme called spermine, and cholesterol are all reduced. PAF is a zinc compound which is highly toxic to most bacteria capable of causing urinary tract infection.

These changes may well affect the quality of semen, and therefore fertility. Certainly it is not uncommon for men with prostatitis to complain that their wives are having difficulty getting pregnant. A sperm count and sperm quality assessment, obtained from a sample of semen following ejaculation, may be used to assess how much a man's fertility is affected if he or his partner are concerned about this.

Treatment

Whenever infection, irritation or allergy involves the prostate gland, inflammation results, causing oedema (swelling). When this process occurs in other parts of the body, the inflammation and swelling gradually subside as the natural resistance of the body and/or medication combat the infection or irritation. The problem in the prostate (and some other parts of the body with a similar drainage system) is different, however. The prostatic duct linings also swell, occluding or partially blocking the ducts. Infected or irritated fluid is retained in millions of tiny microscopic sacs.

Whenever drainage of a closed or partially closed space is restricted, inflammation is difficult to treat and often gets a deeper foothold. In the case of the prostate, it extends through the walls of the tiny glands and finally enters the spaces and tissues between these glands. However, there may be no real correlation between what is going on microscopically and symptoms.

A further problem with drug treatment is that because the organism is not entirely eradicated, it tends to develop immunity to the drug used, and the law of diminishing returns operates. Each time a new medication is tried, improvement may result temporarily, but with subsequently less and less effect.

Unless the prostatitis sufferer understands what the problem is and why his condition is so difficult to 'cure', it may become an obsession with him, as he consults more and more specialists, tries more and more remedies, each time experiencing a 'false dawn' which gives way to relapse and disappointment.

There are however different approaches to the treatment of the different forms of prostatitis, and these are given below.

Urethritis

If this does not extend into the prostate itself, it is normally easily treated with tetracycline or a similar broad-spectrum antibiotic.

CBP

This is usually treated with an antibiotic combination called trimethoprim-sulfamethoxazole (TMP-SMX or Septrin), sometimes for as long as 12 weeks. This usually cures up to half of all sufferers; others may be temporarily cured, but suffer a later relapse, usually caused by the same infective organism. Other antibiotics used for the treatment of CBP include minocycline, doxycycline, carbenicillin, ciprofloxacin and metacycline. In China, trimethoprim has been combined with rifaprim with a reported 80 per cent success rate. In general, choice of antibiotic should be based on the sensitivity of the infecting bacteria.

Other treatments that have been tried on a small scale, with apparent success, include the thrice-daily injection of a large dose of an antibiotic called kanamycin for up to two weeks, and the direct injection of antimicrobial agents such as gentamicin into the prostate through the perineum, which has been tried with apparent success by urologists as far apart as Belgium and China.

Men with CBP not cured by intensive treatment can try continuous suppressive treatment with low-dose medication. The usual drugs are TMP-SMX or nitrofurantoin. These control symptoms and prevent infection of the urine developing, but if the treatment is discontinued the infection is likely to flare up again.

In desperation, some men may ask for prostatectomy in the belief that this will rid them of prostatitis. When a prostatectomy is done (usually because of obstruction caused by benign enlargement), it does sometimes cure the prostatitis as well, but unfortunately this cannot be counted on, and it may even make it worse. The infecting organisms are found in the peripheral parts of the prostate, adjoining the capsule. In TUR, the surgeon has to leave the capsule (only 1–2 mm thick) and probably some compressed prostate tissue intact, and often the infection persists in this tissue. Some urologists will recommend the operation if there are known to be infected calculi, which will be removed during the operation.

NBP

NBP is difficult to treat because although the high white cell count provides evidence of some infection or allergy, the actual infective agent is unknown. In some cases, treatment with tetracyclines seems to bring results, but it is probably only short-lived. TUR is unlikely to cure men with NBP, and should be avoided unless necessary for concurrent benign enlargement.

Treatment with drugs to reduce inflammation and swelling have sometimes proved useful. One group of urologists had good results when they introduced dimethyl sulphoxide, an anti-inflammatory agent, into the urethra, but the treatment is long and has to be repeated. Home treatment with ibuprofen (Nurofen), a non-prescription drug which is anti-inflammatory as well as a painkiller, is sometimes effective.

Prostatodynia

This is a tiresome complaint which is particularly difficult to treat because there is no evidence of any infecting organism, and the patient usually has no history of urinary tract disease. Sufferers complain of pain in the perineum, lower abdomen, testicles, groin or penis, have pain on ejaculating or urinating, and may occasionally have painful erections and low semen volumes. Usually, their urine flow will be abnormally slow, even in the absence of prostatic enlargement, and they have always had difficulty urinating in a public place, according to Graham Watson who runs a prostatitis clinic at the London Institute of Urology.

Many men with prostatodynia are anxious about their condition, even obsessed with it, and go to considerable lengths to track down new treatments or specialists who may be able to hold out some hope of a cure. It is possible that some cases of prostatodynia may be a prostatic variant of a tension headache.

Certainly, in some patients the pain is caused by tension and spasms of the pelvic floor muscles, and these cases are sometimes improved by muscle relaxants such as diazepam (Valium), combined with special exercises and physiotherapy.

These spasms can prevent the urethral (external) sphincter opening properly on urination, causing reflux of urine into the prostate; this may in turn set up an inflammation of the prostate, which makes matters worse. These men, too, may be helped by tranquillizers such as diazepam, and relaxation therapy.

In other men, tension may affect the bladder neck sphincter and muscles of the prostate, resulting in slow urine flow, frequency, getting up in the night, and other symptoms of obstruction. These men respond best to treatment with an alpha-blocking agent, such as Prazosin, whose effect is described in Chapter 5 on page 88. In fact, Graham Watson believes that this drug works better than diazepam in most cases of muscular tension.

Other sufferers may have both pelvic floor myalgia (muscle pain) and a bladder neck or urethral spasm syndrome, in which case prazosin can be combined with diazepam.

Some men with prostatodynia and NBP are clinically neurotic, displaying obsessive and hyper-anxious behaviour. Whether this state is the cause or effect of their prostate problems is often not clear. Typically, they will have consulted many doctors and specialists about their condition, and received varying diagnoses and treatments. Symptoms persist, and the patients become increasingly dissatisfied with medical care. They tend to develop hypochondria, becoming convinced that their condition is more serious than it really is, and often that they are developing cancer.

A good doctor can help by taking time to explain what the condition is and what it is not, providing informed reassurance, and explaining that it is not a critical disease and will not lead to impotence or cancer.

Diazepam may help these patients too, by lowering their general anxiety levels. And where emotional problems and stress seem significant, referral to a psychiatrist for evaluation and treatment is appropriate.

Some NBP and prostatodynia may sometimes be made worse by engorgement of the prostate caused by lack of sexual activity.

It can happen that symptoms flare up, or are first noticed, when there is a change in a man's sexual behaviour, perhaps following the start of a new or break-up of an old relationship.

Many urologists often recommend that sufferers from these two complaints increase the frequency of ejaculation by intercourse or masturbation, because it is thought that one reason for a patient's symptoms is a prostate that has become fluid-laden because of infrequent ejaculations. As well as emptying the prostatic ducts, orgasm also leads to a temporary increase in the blood supply to the prostate, which can lead to a flushing out of the infecting organism. But in some cases, it makes matters worse.

Prostatic massage can also be used to empty the gland of its secretions, although it seems an unnecessary and unpleasant alternative unless the man is unable to ejaculate on his own. However, it does undoubtedly benefit some men.

Often, 'non-medical' treatment to allay symptoms is more help than any drugs. Half an hour in a hot bath or sitz-bath can relieve pelvic floor spasm and improve circulation to the area of the prostate and urethra. In Germany, urologists attach great importance to keeping the prostate area warm, if necessary by wrapping a special 'prostate warmer' between the legs. Regular exercise and bowel movements are recommended, especially for men in sedentary occupations.

Diet does not appear to influence symptoms in most cases, but occasionally sensitivity to alcohol, caffeine or certain foods seems to trigger attacks, and a diary checklist may help to identify an allergy-causing substance.

Among newer treatments, which have been written up in the medical literature but are not yet widely available or internationally accepted, a couple are perhaps worth mentioning: hyperthermia and laser acupuncture therapy. However, it should be stressed that prostatitis can have a very high placebo response – that is, spontaneous improvement takes place when dummy treatment is given – a reminder of the psychosomatic factor in some types of prostatitis. In some studies, the placebo response has been as high as 60 per cent.

The Prostathermer microwave *hyperthermia* delivery system described in Chapter 5 has also been successfully used for the treatment of chronic prostatitis. Israeli urologists have described a significant success rate in treating stubborn cases of chronic prostatitis which have failed to respond to conventional treatment.

Treatment is similar to that given for benign enlargement as described in Chapter 5, with one hour's session of hyperthermia given transrectally once a week for six weeks. Most of the CBP cases were much improved, with white blood cell counts in prostatic fluid near normal after treatment, and pain and obstructive symptoms relieved. NBC and prostatodynia cases have also benefited. Follow-up suggests that these improvements are more than just a remission of symptoms, but more scientific work needs to be done before this procedure is made generally available. It is under trial in both the United Kingdom and the United States, but has yet to receive official approval. It is likely to be available privately in Britain by the time this book appears, but, partly because of the expense of the equipment, will probably not be provided by the National Health Service for some time yet.

As far as its mode of action is understood, hyperthermia, which involves raising the temperature within the prostate from blood heat (37°C) to 42.5°C, increases the blood supply and causes a temporary inflammatory reaction, which may have the effect of increasing the body's natural capacity to deal with the infection or inflammation. Graham Watson (see page 110) thinks that it may also have an action similar to that induced by Prazosin (but more permanent) in relaxing tense muscles, since many men see an improvement in their flow rates.

There have been some suggestions that traditional Chinese

acupuncture therapy is effective in cases of chronic prostatitis, but the work has been mainly done in China, and so far little scientific information on the results has reached the West.

However, a considerable amount of work has been done in the West, the Soviet Union and China on the medical applications of laser beams, and the treatment described below has perhaps more to do with lasers than acupuncture.

It is generally accepted that lasers, as well as having uses in surgery as cutting, cauterizing and joining tools, can be used as a source of irradiation. The helium-neon (HeNe) laser normally used for this purpose can produce anti-inflammatory, painkilling and vasodilatory (blood-vessel-enlarging) effects. Laser irradiation has been used directly through the rectum by Russian urologists to treat chronic inflammation of the prostate.

It has been known for some years that the HeNe laser beam, which is capable of penetrating tissue, can be used in acupuncture as a 'light needle' instead of the traditional metal needle. Chinese medical experts in Shandong Province have combined HeNe laser irradiation with the channel theory of traditional Chinese medicine to treat chronic prostatitis.

Over 100 men were treated with HeNe laser beams channelled through a light-conducting fibre inserted through a tubular acupuncture needle. The laser needle was inserted into the Hui-Ying acupuncture point, situated in the centre of the perineum, between the anus and the scrotum, so as to penetrate into the prostate. Irradiation was given for 15 to 20 minutes, once a day for four days; patients were given one or two courses of treatment, depending on the severity of their prostatitis.

Irradiation with the HeNe laser is non-destructive. This so-called 'mid-laser' improves circulation to the area treated and is also believed to stimulate the immune system; together these two effects could help resolve inflammatory and infectious lesions in the prostate.

The results, reported in the British journal *Laser Therapy* in 1989, were impressive: 55 per cent of the men treated were described as 'fully cured', with clinical symptoms completely abolished and normal white cell count in the prostate fluid, and another 44 per cent were 'improved', with symptoms improved and no evident inflammatory changes in the prostate fluid. Only one man out of 114 showed no improvement at all.

The Chinese team treated another group of patients with direct laser irradiation to the rectum, according to the technique described by the Russian urologists, but the results were less good, with no 'complete cure' reported. However, to discourage eager readers from jumping on the next plane to China, it should be stressed that this study did not include follow-up, so there is no guarantee that these men did not suffer a later relapse.

Living with a chronic condition

It does seem that the best strategy for sufferers from chronic prostatitis is to come to terms with their complaint: it is not crippling or life-threatening, it does not lead to cancer or kidney damage, but it is probably incurable.

It is a chronic condition, like arthritis (inflammation of the joints) or bursitis (inflammation of the cartilage between joints), and like them it cannot be cured but its symptoms can be treated. It comes and goes, and many men are free from symptoms for much of the time. Unlike arthritis, it is not progressive. If your symptoms seem to be linked to uncontrollable tension or anxiety, psychotherapy, perhaps combined with tranquillizers for a time, can probably be of help.

Case history 6.1

Peter S., from Cornwall, is 51 and has had chronic prostatitis for many years. 'I have constant pain in the prostate and also acute pain on ejaculation. After suffering this for several years, and having repeated doses of antibiotic without any effect, and seeing consultants in Cornwall and Oxford, all I am being offered now is surgery or pain management. I feel that surgery is too drastic a measure for what is really chronic inflammation, and as for pain management, I have been coping with pain by myself for years. But the constant pain is debilitating, and I never feel really well.'

Case history 6.2

Arthur K., an American living in Paris, developed symptoms of prostatitis when in his mid-50s. He saw a urologist, who told him he had benign enlargement as well, and gave him antibiotics. But the prostatitis kept coming back, with discomfort, burning and tenderness. 'Over the last three years it has made my life a misery – not all the time, but a lot of the time. The irritation causes premature ejaculation – my sex life is ruined! All the consultant can say is that semen is bland and neutral and shouldn't cause burning – but it does. He says he can do nothing more for me, and even a prostatectomy will not necessarily get rid of the symptoms.'

Case history 6.3

Richard T., a senior Royal Air Force officer, was struck down with prostatitis out of the blue while serving in the British Embassy in Washington. 'On a driving holiday with my wife and children, somewhere in the remote Mid-West, my left testicle became painful and swelled up. Fortunately it improved in a day or two, and when I got back to Washington I went to the Herbert Reed Hospital to be checked over. They told me it was prostatitis (although I had no pain in that region) and that the pain was "transferred" to the testicle. Antibiotics cleared up the original infection and the swelling, but the pain in the testicle has kept recurring since.'

CHAPTER 7

What alternative and complementary medicine have to offer

Do 'alternative' treatments, diets and supplements have any effect on prostate problems? Men anxious to avoid prostate surgery, or those faced with a long wait for a 'non-urgent' operation, may be tempted to try out a variety of alternative treatments for their problem, especially if they have used these successfully for other ailments in the past.

Of course, had any of these treatments shown a remarkable success, with results backed up by serious scientific research, the world – and prostate sufferers – would no doubt know all about it. In the absence of such certainties, a question-mark must remain about how useful such therapies may be.

Benign prostate enlargement and prostatitis are both quite variable conditions whose symptoms sometimes change from day to day. Because of this, complementary medical practitioners and their patients find it difficult to evaluate whether or not their various treatments are truly successful. Scientific trials with experimental drugs have shown that up to 30 per cent of prostate sufferers with benign enlargement will claim an improvement in their symptoms when they are just given a placebo (dummy pill); and with some forms of prostatitis, the placebo response is sometimes as high as 60 per cent. In these circumstances it is not difficult to find a herbal potion or a procedure which can 'benefit' a sizeable proportion of sufferers.

All branches of alternative and complementary medicine claim, with varying degrees of confidence, to be able to cure benign enlargement and prostatitis. Some claim that attention to diet, lifestyle and posture will prevent disease developing in the first place. There is little doubt that some of these claims are at least partially justified, and equally that some of them are pretty worthless.

What should the bewildered prostate sufferer think? If he asks his doctor or consultant whether it would be worth his trying this or that diet or remedy, he will almost inevitably be told not to waste his money. On the other hand, he may think, probably rightly, that the treatment can do him no harm, so he has little to lose.

There are certain areas of alternative medicine where proper scientific trials are carried out and which thereby acquire an aura of 'respectability' in the eyes of at least part of the traditional medical establishment. A good example of this is the laser acupuncture treatment for chronic prostatitis developed in China and described in Chapter 6. This particular type of treatment – the irradiation by the heat and light of a laser beam – is one where conventional and alternative experimental treatments have converged, since interstitial laser irradiation of the prostate is being tested at this very moment in both the United States and Britain for the treatment of benign enlargement. The process used is very similar to that used by the Chinese: the laser beams are introduced through hollow needles inserted into the prostate through the perineum, although the type of laser used is quite different and has different effects.

It is areas like this, where some scientific results have been published, which offer the best hope for the prostate sufferer eager to try out less conventional treatment for his complaint. He should however be extremely wary of any treatment claiming to 'cure' benign enlargement, and recall that if a reliable cure was known, in any branch of medicine, those cured would proclaim it from the rooftops.

Such proclamations being conspicuously absent, this chapter will be mainly restricted to a bare description of the treatments on offer – there are other publications already available which deal with them in more detail – with closer attention being paid to a few areas which have some proven scientific respectability.

Lifestyle

It is undeniable that a healthy diet and lifestyle are likely to make most people feel better, have a better resistance to infections – probably even live longer. If you do not smoke, you are statistically less likely to contract cancer of the lung or bladder and certain other diseases; if you do not drink too much alcohol, you are less likely to contract liver disease or cancer of the oesophagus.

But there are few provable direct links between lifestyle and prostate disease. Prostate cancer does not seem to be one of those made more likely by smoking. Benign enlargement is not made more probable by excessive or restricted sexual activity. There *is* an association between sexually transmitted disease and some forms of prostatitis, but it is not a clear-cut one.

Alcohol

Because it is a central nervous system depressant, and reduces muscle tone generally throughout the body, alcohol does have an effect on bladder function. Even men without prostate enlargement may fail to empty their bladder completely after drinking a lot of alcohol, so it is not surprising that men with outflow obstruction are more likely to have chronic retention if they habitually drink a lot of alcohol, and are also more likely to have an episode of acute retention. This will require immediate medical attention and catheterization, and will probably lead to them being put on the list for prostatectomy, since many urologists believe that an episode of acute retention is a convincing indication for surgery.

By the same token, a man who lives healthily, with plenty of fresh air and exercise, and a good diet and little or no alcohol, is likely to have better general muscle tone and to empty his bladder more efficiently than a man who leads a sedentary existence, with a regular high alcohol intake.

Diet

Dieticians tell us that we should all eat foods high in fibre, low in cholesterol and saturated fats, and including plenty of fresh fruit and vegetables. Such a diet will improve bowel health and should reduce blood cholesterol levels, and men with benign enlargement will benefit from both these factors. They may also find it best to avoid spicy foods and coffee, as both these substances can increase bladder irritability. It is also important to avoid drinking more than small amounts of alcohol, because, as explained above, alcohol reduces the efficiency of the bladder muscles and encourages retention of urine.

A man with chronic constipation will find this condition worsened by prostate enlargement, because the enlarged prostate may press against the rectum and make it more difficult to pass a hard stool. Constipation can also worsen prostate problems, because hard stools pressing against the prostate can further retard the flow of urine. A healthy diet, with plenty of fruit and vegetable fibre or bran, can reduce or eliminate this problem.

Research has shown that enlarged prostate tissue contains raised levels of cholesterol, but although there have been attempts to treat benign enlargement by lowering blood cholesterol, these have not had very convincing results. Of course, lowering raised blood cholesterol levels can do nothing but good, and some practitioners claim that the process leads to an improvement in prostate symptoms, if not size.

Sugar, fats, and too much meat and dairy produce should also be avoided, according to naturopathic experts. It certainly seems probable that Western diets, with high fat, sugar and meat content, do lead to hormonal imbalance as well as an increased level of heart disease. Since both benign enlargement and prostate cancer are known to be hormone-dependent diseases, there may well be something in these theories. In fact, in China and Japan prostate cancer is less common (see Chapter 8), and it has been suggested that this is due to local diet, which is low in fat and rich in green and yellow vegetables (vitamins A and C). Whether dietary improvements will help cure the disease, or arrest its development, once it has begun, is another question.

Supplements

Naturopaths claim that some dietary supplements can prevent and even cure prostate disease. The main supplements proposed are essential fatty acids (EFAs) and other vitamins, amino acids, and zinc.

As far as zinc is concerned, two things have been known for

many years: that zinc is essential to human growth and development, and that zinc is concentrated in the prostate and in semen. It seems that zinc concentrations in semen and the prostate fall in the presence of prostate disease, particularly prostatitis. Some dieticians claim that taking zinc supplements will improve symptoms, but this has not been proved to the satisfaction of conventional medicine. It is also suggested by naturopaths that a deficiency of zinc increases the production of DHT, the hormone believed to be responsible for benign enlargement, by increasing the activity of 5-alpha reductase, the enzyme that converts testosterone to DHT.

Zinc is present in many common foods, and some foods, such as oysters and herrings, are particularly rich in it, possibly lending credence to the theory of the aphrodisiac properties of oysters. Oatmeal, wheat bran, milk, peas and nuts are among several foods which contain useful amounts.

Obviously, it is not a good thing to be deficient in zinc, whether or not your prostate or sex life suffer because of it. People on a balanced diet are unlikely to be, but a simple tasting test, available from health food shops, will enable you to check whether you need a supplement.

Essential fatty acids (EFAs) are also important for health. Also known as vitamin F, EFAs are useful to the body in many ways, combating cholesterol and helping to metabolize saturated fats. The most important EFA is linoleic acid, good sources of which are safflower seed oil, evening primrose oil, sunflower seed oil and linseed oil. Most prominent in health food stores are Evening Primrose Oil capsules, which also contain important gammalinolenic acid. If enough linoleic acid is present in the diet, the body can itself manufacture the other EFAs. Some studies have suggested that EFA supplements can help benign enlargement, but again conventional medical specialists are unconvinced.

Other vitamins, notably E and C, are recommended as supplements for prostate sufferers. Some naturopaths suggest that a high-protein diet protects against prostate disease, and that modern man can conveniently imitate the effects of that by taking amino acid supplements: three specific substances are mentioned as particularly important among the 20 or so that exist – glycine, glutamic acid and alanine.

None of these supplements can do any harm when taken in sensible doses. Naturopaths tend to recommend most or all of them, claiming that some help others work better. Thus the American naturopathic guru, Dr Kurt Donsbach, who runs a clinic in Baja California, Mexico, recommends the following daily supplements for prostate sufferers:

- A handful of pumpkin seeds
- Four tablespoons food-grade flaxseed oil
- Multi-vitamin tablets plus zinc
- Amino acids
- Nine tablets of chlorophyll extract
- Forty drops of 35 per cent food grade hydrogen peroxide
- Twenty-four ounces of cranberry juice.

The 'grapeshot' nature of this prescription may suggest simply that not much confidence is placed in any single supplement. Undoubtedly, much naturopathic theorizing is made suspect by the fact that so many remedies are prescribed simultaneously. Admittedly, individuals and their bodies differ, and what may benefit one man may leave another unchanged – this certainly applies to conventional drug treatment as well.

But until more serious scientific studies are done – and these unfortunately cost money – the prostate sufferer can only be advised to apply his common sense to what he is told, and keep his sense of proportion – and sense of humour. If you have been medically assessed, and are 'under observation', then clearly diets and supplements can do no harm, and may conceivably do good. The danger comes if you rely on them as a cure, especially if not under medical supervision, because the bladder and kidneys can suffer irreversible damage when urine is chronically retained.

Homoeopathy and plant extracts

While homoeopathic treatment of some diseases, such as rheumatoid arthritis and fibrositis, seems successful in many cases, it must be said that homoeopathy does not have much to offer to the prostate sufferer with serious outflow problems. However, some plant extracts are of undoubted benefit in some cases, and a few are accepted by conventional urologists.

Many conventional drugs derive, or derived originally, from

plant extracts. Famous cases are belladonna, reserpine, digitalis and the contraceptive pill (derived from a plant hormone present in the Mexican yam). In France, Italy and Germany drugs made from plant extracts are much more commonly used than in the English-speaking world: often they are prescribed by conventional doctors and urologists, and their cost reimbursed by the health insurance schemes or social security. Few, however, are available in the United Kingdom or United States.

Like conventional pharmaceutical drugs, these pills can theoretically improve prostate symptoms in a number of different ways. They can shrink or soften the gland so that it presses less on the urethra. They can relax the muscles of the prostate and the bladder neck so that urination becomes easier. They can reduce the irritability of the obstructed bladder, thus improving symptoms of urgency and frequency. Or they can improve the tone of the bladder muscle, leading to better voiding. This is the theory: in practice, naturopathic products, with one possible exception, are unlikely to be able to do more than reduce bladder irritability – improving symptoms, but doing nothing to relieve their cause.

Among medicines commonly available in Europe are those derived from stinging nettle root, golden rod (*Solidago*) flowers, *Pygeum africanum* (a type of African plum), and the fruit of the saw palmetto (*Serenoa repens*). Stinging nettle extract is claimed to inhibit the binding of hormones to the receptors in the prostate, which could quite possibly help to relieve or contain the process of benign enlargement (the proprietary extract is called Bazoton). The African plum extract (marketed in France under the brand name Tadenan) is supposed to have a similar function. But the saw palmetto is probably the most interesting plant for treating prostate disease, because it appears to have an influence on the mechanism of benign enlargement of the prostate rather similar to that of the new drugs currently under development by leading pharmaceutical companies to inhibit the production of dihydro-testosterone (DHT) in the prostate.

The saw palmetto (see Fig. 7.1) is a small palm tree native to the Atlantic Coast of North America from South Carolina to Florida, growing up to 10 feet high with a crown of large leaves. The dark reddish-brown berries of the palm were used by the American Indians and later by naturopaths and homoeopaths to treat genito-urinary tract disturbances.

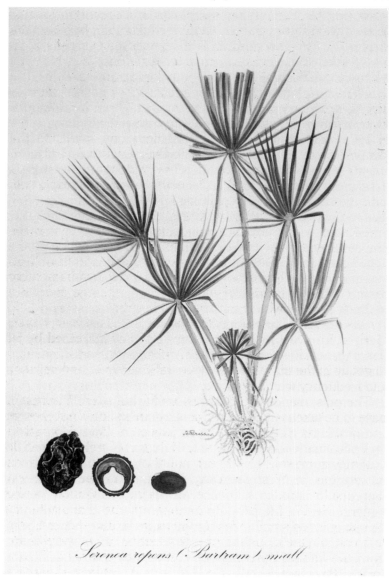

Serenoa repens (Bartram) small

Photograph courtesy of Fabre SA

Fig. 7.1: saw palmetto

For many years homoeopaths, who also know the plant by another Latin name, *Sabal serruta,* have reported its efficacy in improving bladder outflow symptoms. But recently scientific studies have shown that an oil derived from the berries, containing saturated and unsaturated fatty acids and sterols, actually prevents the conversion of testosterone to DHT (the hormone responsible for benign enlargement) and inhibits the binding of DHT to receptor sites in the prostate, thereby increasing the breakdown and excretion of DHT. In addition to this anti-androgen effect, the extract also appears to have properties which reduce oedema (swelling) and stimulate the immune system. This is a dramatic discovery: as described in Chapter 5 (where the action of 5-alpha reductase inhibitors is explained more fully), two of the world's largest pharmaceutical companies have been spending hundreds of millions of dollars in attempts to synthesize drugs with a similar action.

A French pharmaceutical company produces pills containing the specific lipo-sterolic extract of *Serenoa* which is the active ingredient, and a number of scientific studies have been carried out, mainly in France and Italy, which show impressive results in patients with benign enlargement. In several trials in which these pills were compared to other pills or placebos, the results compared favourably to those obtained in trials of other non-surgical treatments. Flow rates typically increased by 50 per cent, residual urine and the number of times patients had to get up in the night were substantially reduced, and urgency and frequency were improved.

The pills, marketed in Europe under the name Permixon, have to be taken on a regular basis, but this should not present any problems as they have been proved to have a complete lack of toxicity. In France alone, more than a million monthly treatments are sold every year, and the pills are widely taken in Italy too. In West Germany, Permixon is one of the few naturopathic products to receive official recognition by the Federal Health Ministry. Unfortunately, the manufacturing company is too small to justify the expense and risk of trying to break into the British or American markets, but the pills are available without a prescription in most pharmacies in France (price 105 francs for 15 days' treatment). Interested readers may enquire about the possibility of obtaining the pills outside France to: Dr Michel Sestier, Laboratoires Fabre SA, 192 rue Lecourbe, F–75015 Paris, telephone (+331) 45.30.19.79.

Those able to obtain them may try eating the fruit of the saw palmetto itself: quite a small quantity of the berries – about 20g a day – should provide a dose of the active ingredient equivalent to that provided by the pills, the daily dose of which provides 320mg of the serolipid extract. Homoeopathic pharmacies sell a tincture of the whole fruit, and some naturopaths suggest 20 drops of this extract three times a day. This is worth trying, in the absence of the pills, although it provides a lower dose, and large doses of the extract should be avoided as it is alcohol-based.

Turning now to more physical methods, the German-speaking world has a particular proliferation of alternative prostate treatments (although this did not prevent Chancellor Helmut Kohl from having a conventional TUR in 1989). One of the most surprising, sounding as though it belongs more to the 18th-century theories of galvanism than to the end of the 20th century, is treatment by electro-magnets.

Magnetic field therapy

The claims made for this therapy, which involves placing a south-pole applicator in the rectum and a north-pole applicator over the abdomen, are extravagant, with a 'total cure rate' of 70 per cent, apparently for both benign enlargement and prostatitis. A high-intensity magnetic field is generated, of 10–50 Gauss, with a frequency of 8–10 Hertz. The treatment must however be given with care, as the north-pole magnetic field can affect the nerves and arterial system of the penis, causing impotence. (Should this happen, the effect can apparently be reversed by appropriate application of the south-pole field.)

Treatment is given once or twice weekly for a maximum of six weeks and should be accompanied by homoeopathic medicine and a special diet.

Neural therapy

Also practised in Germany, this therapy consists of injecting the prostate gland through the perineum with 4–5ml of local anaesthetic such as procain, impletol or xyloneurol. It is not clear what effect this therapy is intended to have or how often it needs to be repeated. It seems likely to cause infection if not done with scrupulous care.

British urologists have tried giving injections of a substance including glacial acetic acid and phenol, designed to shrivel the gland. Given through a large-gauge needle, the injections worked in some cases, but caused problems in other cases, and the experiments were discontinued.

Reflex massage

This is a type of compression massage originating, like acupuncture, in China, and using a similar system of 'reflex points'. Practitioners claim to be able to relieve the symptoms of urinary obstruction caused by benign enlargement. When prostate disease is present, two main reflex areas become sensitive and can be massaged: the first is on the outer thigh, about a third of the way between the hip and knee; and the second is at the base of the spine. Pressure applied to these points is thought to reduce lymphatic congestion in the area of the prostate. No one claims that the result is a cure, but treatment may result in symptomatic relief of prostatitis and benign enlargement.

Acupuncture

Acupuncturists claim to be able to relieve the symptoms of prostatitis and benign enlargement, and some scientific papers have been published to support this. Some cases of prostatitis being cured are given, although long-term follow-up is lacking. No cure of benign enlargement is claimed.

Bio-feedback

This is a system of bodily control not unlike meditation. Its aim is to make the person aware of bodily processes and enable them to have some influence over unconscious or vegetative bodily processes such as pulse, blood pressure, digestion or bowel function. Electrical apparatus can be provided to help the person be more aware of various bodily functions.

It can be useful in prostatitis and benign enlargement, mainly in improving bladder control. At its basic level, everyone can use bio-feedback to be aware of when his bladder has been fully emptied. When the bladder empties completely, there is a certain almost pleasurable sensation of relief, which men with benign enlargement and some types of prostatitis can forget the existence of. The reassurance that complete emptying has occurred which bio-feedback can provide is valuable to the man who tends to worry constantly about his condition.

If a partially obstructed man is in a hurry. or doesn't bother to ask himself whether his bladder has emptied properly, the chances are that it will not empty. This will leave a vague feeling of dissatisfaction and mean that he will need to go again sooner than he should. Relaxation is essential for good emptying.

Another factor which may be relevant is that unlike women, men urinate standing up – an 'unnatural' posture for the function. Try sitting or squatting, or sitting then standing – and don't be hurried. Once you identify the feeling of emptiness, cultivate it and make sure that you achieve it every time. Providing you are emptying your bladder completely, no harm can come to your kidneys – and this is always the most important consideration in prostate enlargement. But remember that chronic retention can build up gradually, and it is important to have regular medical supervision once you have developed prostate problems.

CHAPTER 8

Prostate cancer: incidence, diagnosis and treatment

Adenocarcinoma of the prostate, as the cancer is technically called, is one of the commoner cancers. In the United Kingdom, it is the third most commonly occurring cancer in men (after lung cancer and skin cancer), and the second most common cause of male cancer death (if colon and rectal cancer deaths are counted separately). In the latest year for which figures are available, there were over 10,800 new cases and over 7,500 deaths. In the United States, some 100,000 new cases are diagnosed, and over 26,000 men die of it, every year; it accounts for about 20 per cent of all cancer deaths in males in that country.

It is thus a bigger killer in men than cervical cancer is in women, yet we read much less about it and there are few suggestions that men should be screened for it. There are reasons for this, the main ones being that prostate cancer affects an older age group than cervical cancer, and also that it is more difficult to detect and less easy to cure: there is nothing equivalent to a Pap smear. When it spreads outside the prostate, it usually affects the lymph nodes, and then the bones, and at that point becomes virtually incurable.

Like the other diseases of the prostate, prostate cancer behaves strangely in many respects. Of all the common human cancers, its causes are probably the least well understood: it has no clear connection with diet, drink, smoking or environmental factors, Although some recent studies have suggested that vasectomized men are more likely to develop the disease. Curiously, men of some races seem more likely to develop it than others.

Incidence

Yet there are huge variations in the incidence of prostate cancer between ethnic groups and geographic locations. The
highest incidence is in North America and Scandinavia, and
the lowest in the Far East. Intermediate rates are reported
from England, France and Italy, while rates from the Balkan
countries and Israel are relatively lower. But within the United States itself there are surprising differences: for instance,
the rate for blacks living in Detroit is nearly double that for
whites living in the same city. Yet this difference does not
seem to be linked to differences in prosperity between the
two groups.

Yet while US blacks have a very high incidence, blacks living in West Africa, who are genetically similar, have a very low

USA, California, Alameda		Denmark	23.6
County, blacks	100.2	UK, Scotland, North-East	23.4
USA, Michigan, Detroit,		Italy, Varese	22.8
blacks	73.2	USA, California, Los	
USA, Georgia, Atlanta,		Angeles County, Japanese	21.5
whites	51.9	Spain, Zaragoza	20.7
Sweden	44.4	Cuba	19.9
USA, Hawaii, Hawaiian	42.5	UK, England and Wales,	
USA, Michigan, Detroit,		Mersey region	18.1
whites	41.4	Germany, Dresden	18.1
New Zealand, Maori	39.8	Spain, Navarra	17.6
Australia, South Australia	39.6	Yugoslavia, Slovenia	15.8
Norway	38.9	Israel, Jews	15.5
USA, Hawaii, Japanese	35.9	Poland, Warsaw City	14.6
Germany, Saarland	32.9	Japan, Nagasaki City	10.2
USA, New Mexico,		Romania, County Cluj	9.7
American Indian	31.6	Czechoslovakia, Western	
New Zealand, Non-Maori	30.7	Slovakia	8.1
Jamaica, Kingston and St		Singapore, Malay	7.2
Andrew	28.6	India, Bombay	6.8
Finland	27.2	Hong Kong	5.1
USA, California, Los		Singapore, Chinese	4.8
Angeles County, Chinese	26.6	Africa, Senegal, Dakar	4.3
France, Doubs	25.7		

Fig. 8.1: incidence of prostate cancer per 100,000 males

incidence, although this is at least partly due to smaller proportions of elderly men there and above all to poorer diagnosis. And Japanese men living in the United States are three or four times as likely to develop the disease as native Japanese, who have one of the lowest rates in the world.

One factor that has been associated with the low incidence of prostate cancer in Japan and China is the high consumption of green and yellow vegetables - nearly three times that in the USA - and it has been suggested that it is the high content of vitamins A and C in the Japanese diet which protects against prostate cancer. But the evidence is circumstantial, and the genetic factor seems likely to be more important.

Post-mortem evidence suggests that these wide variations are not so much in true incidence, but in the development of clinical disease from cancer which is commonly present anyway. The difference thus lies more in the effectiveness of the body's immunological response in keeping the disease at bay.

Contrary to what might be expected, social factors do not seem to have much influence on prostate cancer incidence. A study by the British Office of Population Censuses and Surveys, published in 1990, suggests that while British people are more likely to die of most other cancers if they are poor, this is not the case for prostate cancer. The study compared the death rates from cancers registered between 1971 and 1981 among middle-class people who owned their own homes with those among council tenants.

For most cancers, the poorer people had a higher death rate, probably because their cancers were not diagnosed so early as those of middle-class people, who make better use of the health services. Prostate cancer was one of the only cancers for which middle-class people had a higher mortality rate. This may be because the middle-class men tended to live longer and so were more likely to develop the disease.

Again, unlike most other cancers, prostate cancer often exists in elderly men without being evident or causing any symptoms, and as men get older, the more likely they are to have the latent disease. The incidence of latent cancer increases in each decade and is found in about 70 per cent of men over 80. Yet less than half of 1 per cent of these cancers ever cause problems. Certainly, men over 70 with prostate cancer are five times as likely to die with it than because of it.

To illustrate the vast scale of the disease in its undetected form, it is estimated that at any one time there are at least 5 million men in the United States alone with latent prostate cancer; of these, only half (2.5 million) will ever show clinical evidence of the disease, and only 13 per cent (650,000) will actually die of it. These estimates are used by those urologists who argue against mass screening for the disease, for even if, they reason, the screening detected all 5 million cases, 87 per cent of those would be treated unnecessarily and would be adversely affected by the necessary therapy. However, the incidence of latent cancer is not known with any certainty, particularly in the younger age groups, for which little post-mortem evidence is available. The pros and cons of screening are further discussed in Chapter 9.

One thing that is known for certain about the cancer is that it is a disease of old age. It is virtually unknown in men under 45, and its incidence increases in direct proportion to ageing, which may be because the body's immunological response declines with age. Longer life expectancy thus carries with it an increased incidence of prostate cancer, and while it is so far predominantly a disease of the rich industrialized countries, it will certainly increasingly be found in the developing world as more men survive to old age there.

Diagnosis

Prostate cancer develops in the outer part of the gland, and most commonly the diagnosis is made by a doctor carrying out a rectal examination. Cancer often changes the consistency of the gland, and forms nodules or irregularities which can easily be felt by the doctor's finger, assuming they are in the part of the gland that he can reach during a rectal examination. Its role as a cancer check is in fact the most useful function of the rectal examination, because the size of the gland does not really tell the doctor very much: a large benign prostate may not be obstructive, a small one still may.

However, up to a half of all men referred to specialists because of 'suspicious' findings in a rectal examination turn out not to have cancer at all: the irregularities turn out to be caused by calculi, benign enlargement, a certain type of prostatitis or other non-malignant changes.

A good number of cases – between 15 and 30 per cent of all those diagnosed – are undetected at rectal examination but are discovered when the tissue removed during a prostatectomy is checked for cancer cells. The only symptoms that early prostate cancer may produce (although it may not do so) are obstructive symptoms similar to those caused by benign enlargement, but probably with a more sudden onset. Almost certainly, it will coexist with benign enlargement.

A technique which is not yet widely available but is likely to be increasingly used for diagnosis in the future is transrectal ultrasound. From the patient's point of view, this is a simple and painless procedure: a lubricated probe, not much thicker than a finger, is placed in the rectum, and the resulting images viewed on a visual display screen and photocopied for reference. But it is an expensive procedure and requires a lot of training, experience and familiarity on the part of the operator before really good results are obtained.

The newer high-resolution ultrasound probes, operating at 7 Mhz, are capable of detecting cancerous lesions which are either too small to be felt by the doctor's finger, or somewhere in the prostate beyond his reach. It can also help determine how far the cancer has spread within the prostate.

Biopsy

When a doctor suspects cancer because of the texture of the prostate at rectal examination or a suspicious rectal ultrasound scan, a biopsy must be done to check that it really is cancer, because this is the only means of confirming the presence of cancer. In Scandinavia and Europe, and increasing in the United States, initial biopsies are mainly done by the 'skinny needle aspiration' technique. This has the advantage over traditional biopsy technique of using a smaller diameter needle, and aspirations can easily be performed in an outpatient setting using only local anaesthesia (see Fig. 8.2).

Core (or Tru-cut) biopsy, which was in general use for years, required general or regional anaesthesia and carried a higher risk of infection when done through the usual rectal route. Fine needle aspiration can provide several samples with minimal bleeding or risk of infection - but it does require the availability of a skilled cytologist to interpret the cores

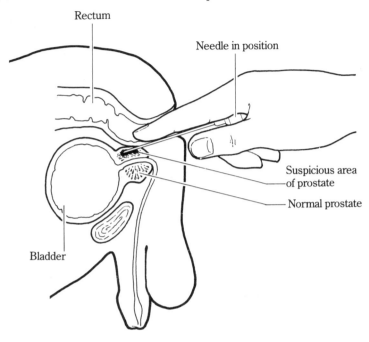

Fig. 8.2: 'skinny-needle' biopsy

obtained. It has also been claimed to be more accurate, with few false positives, as well as cheaper, easier and preferred by the patient. It causes less inflammation and damage to the prostate capsule than core biopsy, which makes a radical prostatectomy (see below), if one should be needed, technically easier. A further use of transrectal ultrasound is to help guide the aspiration or core biopsy needle into suspicious areas of the prostate.

A recent development, which apparently offers advantages to urologist and patient, is endoscopic biopsy. In this procedure, a special spring-loaded core-biopsy needle (called an endocut needle) is passed through a cystoscope, the instrument used to view the interior of the urethra and bladder. The patient is given an injection of a tranquillizer, Midazolam, and his urethra is anaesthetized with lignocaine gel, as for a cystoscopy. A core biopsy of prostate (or bladder) tissue is obtained by firing the needle and retrieving it through the endoscope. The British urologists who developed the tech-

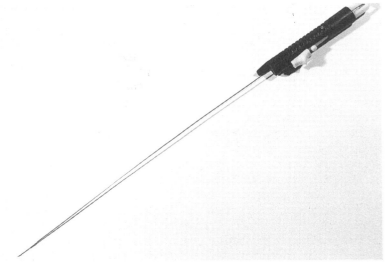

Photograph courtesy of W. CooksLtd

Fig. 8.3: endocut needle

nique claim that the endocut needle provides a less traumatic and more accurate and safe method of prostatic biopsy; there is a much lower rate of infection than for biopsies carried out through the rectum, and what is more, it is preferred by patients who have experienced both methods. It is also believed to avoid entirely the risk of the 'seeding' of cancer outside the prostate which exists with other forms of biopsy.

Staging and grading of the disease

Cancers are diseases of the cells (the building blocks) of the body. Normally, the repair and reproduction of these cells takes place in an orderly and controlled manner, but if, for some reason, the process gets out of control the cells will continue to divide, developing into a lump which is called a tumour.

If the tumour is benign (normal prostatic enlargement is a sort of benign tumour) the cells do not spread to other parts of the body. But a malignant tumour is made up of cells which have the ability to spread beyond the original site, and if left untreated they may invade and destroy surrounding tissues. Sometimes cells break away from the original (primary) tumour and spread to other organs in the body via the bloodstream or lymphatic system. When these cells reach a new site, they may go on dividing and form a new tumour, often referred to as a secondary tumour or 'metastasis'. Cancer cells also have different degrees of malignancy which can be assessed in the laboratory.

So once cancer has been diagnosed, it is important to determine what stage it has reached and what grade of malignancy it has so that appropriate treatment can be given. There are various systems of staging, but they all describe the size and extent of the tumour, the degree of involvement of the pelvic lymph nodes, and the degree of metastasis (the development of new tumours in other parts of the body).

The grading of the tumour is also important. This is done at biopsy, either through a subjective assessment by the pathologist, who assigns what is called a 'Gleason score' from 2 to 10 to the tissue, or sometimes nowadays by an expensive technique called 'flow cytometry', which examines the genetic make-up of individual cells and grades them from 1 to 4 according to their degree of malignancy.

One of the commonly used systems of staging is that devised by the American Urologists Association (AUA). It divides cancers into four stages – A, B, C, D – which can be further subdivided into 1 and 2. Thus Stage A describes the 'occult' stage of prostate cancer in which it cannot be detected by digital examination, and is usually only found by tissue analysis after a prostatectomy for benign enlargement. If there is less than about two cubic centimetres of malignant tumour in the tissue removed, then the cancer is staged A1, and little or no further treatment is usually given. But if the tumour is bigger than this, or appears to be of high-grade malignancy, then it is staged A2 and therapy is needed.

Stage B cancer is more extensive within the prostate and can be detected by digital rectal examination. In Stage C, the cancer is still thought to be restricted to the prostate and accessory glands (seminal vesicles), but is extensive throughout the prostate and involves the capsule. A Stage D cancer is one in which the cancer has spread outside the prostate gland, first to the seminal vesicles and the bladder, then the pelvic lymph nodes, and finally to the bones in the lower part of the body and possibly elsewhere.

There are a number of blood tests which are of limited use for diagnosing the presence or absence of cancer, because of a high proportion of false negatives, but which are very useful to the specialist for staging the disease and monitoring the success of treatment. The main ones used are the prostate acid phosphatase (PAP) test and the prostate-specific antigen (PSA) test. These measure the level in the bloodstream of two substances produced by the prostate in abnormal quantities when cancer is present. The PSA test is the most sensitive, and is particularly useful for checking whether cancer has spread outside the prostate capsule; for instance, if a cancer patient is given a radical prostatectomy (see below), his PSA level should fall to almost zero – if it is still above a certain level, it almost certainly means that the cancer has spread.

The best way of making sure that a cancer which is believed to be confined to the prostate really has not spread, is to carry out a bone scan to look for evidence. This is done by injecting a radioactive material into a vein, which then concentrates in bone tissue, especially where there has been repair and regeneration. The patient is then scanned by a machine which maps the distribution of the radioactive material: increased radioactivity is evidence of cancer or other repairs, such as fractures or arthritis. A negative scan is a strong indication that the cancer has not spread to the bones.

Treatment

Treatment for prostate cancer, except for cancers of the most clear-cut variety, varies widely from country to country and even urologist to urologist. Because of the often unpredictable nature of the disease, there is plenty of room for doubt and argument as to which treatment is likely to cure the cancer, cause a remittance of symptoms, or prolong the patient's life – even as to whether any treatment at all should be given.

It has been said that if a man with prostate cancer goes to four different specialists, he may get four different suggestions for treatment. But this is really only probable in a limited number of cases, when there is uncertainty about the spread of the disease or the patient's life expectancy because he is old or has other diseases.

However, British urologists have been more conservative than those in the United States or many European countries in their attitude to screening for prostate cancer and to aggressive treatment.

There is general agreement that if the cancer is proved to be confined to the prostate, the chances of a cure are good and therapy should aim to achieve this. If the cancer has spread to the prostate capsule and the seminal vesicles, there may still be a chance of curing it, through radiotherapy or radical prostatectomy (see below). But if it has spread further afield, to the bones, it is likely to be incurable, and any therapy should be applied to control the further spread of the cancer and making the symptoms as bearable as possible.

If cancer is detected by chance through rectal examination, and it seems clear that it has not spread outside the prostate, the most likely treatment to be offered is a TUR if there is associated obstruction. This will be performed as thoroughly as possible, to remove all the tissue down to the prostate capsule. Then the man will be asked to come back in a month or two's time, when the prostate has healed, to receive radiotherapy or laser treatment, to attempt to eradicate any remaining cancer cells in the capsule.

Other alternatives are doing nothing – keeping the man under observation, likely if he is very old; radiotherapy; and radical prostatectomy.

Radiotherapy

External beam radiotherapy, that is, bombardment of the prostate area by a beam of radioactive particles like those released by an X-ray machine, is generally used for larger tumours within the prostate. Side-effects of the treatment include diarrhoea, rectal discomfort, painful and frequent urination and blood in the urine. There are doubts over the effectiveness of this approach, since between 35 and 70 per cent of patients still have prostatic tumours 12 months after treatment (although the proportion falls to 20 per cent at 24–30 months), and there is evidence that such men are at increased risk of the cancer spreading outside the prostate.

What is more, about half the patients undergoing radiation therapy for prostate cancer will become impotent as a result of the effects of radiation on the blood vessels supplying the spongy parts of the penis. A minority will also have long-term problems of the bladder or bowel, with extreme urinary frequency or diarrhoea.

On the other hand, even when cancer cells still show on a biopsy after radiation treatment, the treatment may have impaired their malignancy and made them spread at a slower rate.

Interstitial irradiation is sometimes used to treat small, localized prostatic tumours. This involves inserting radioactive iodine 'seed' implants into the cancerous tissue. Again, there is doubt about the effectiveness of this treatment, and side-effects also occur.

Radical prostatectomy

An alternative to this treatment is radical prostatectomy. In this operation, the entire prostate, capsule, seminal vesicles and all, is removed, usually by the retropubic route, and the bladder neck joined directly to the divided urethra close to the external sphincter. It carries increased risks of incontinence and impotence, although a recent nerve-sparing variation of the opera-

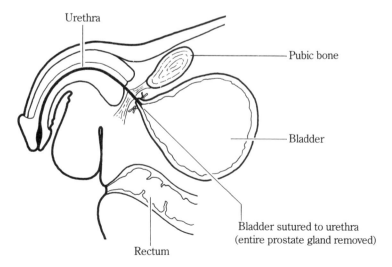

Fig. 8.4: radical prostatectomy

tion now can usually preserve potency.

Before the operation proper begins, the surgeon usually removes the pelvic lymph nodes and has them examined to see whether or not the cancer has spread to them. It is important to know this, and some urologists will only go ahead with a radical prostatectomy if the cancer is shown not to have spread outside the prostate, as the operation is a very long one, taking two to four hours, with a long convalescence. It is not usually thought to be worth submitting a man to this operation if his cancer has already spread.

Radical prostatectomy is favoured in the United States, especially for treatment of the younger patient who may have 20 years or more of life expectancy if his cancer is cured. It is also widely carried out in West Germany and Austria, and increasingly in France and Italy. Urologists in Britain have tended to shun it, although now that the nerve-sparing operation has proved its success, many of the younger surgeons are increasingly interested in its life-saving possibilities. The operation is still little performed in Britain; for instance, in Scotland in 1988, when some 1,200 new cases of prostate cancer were diagnosed, not a single radical prostatectomy was carried out. Many US urologists would find this incredible, but part of the explanation is that many British prostate cancer cases are diagnosed too late for the operation to be of value.

Hormone therapy

Once prostatic cancer has spread beyond the gland itself, the aim of treatment is to control rather than cure the disease. Since the growth of prostate cancer is dependent on levels of circulating male hormones, principally testosterone, it has been common practice to attempt to reduce the levels of these hormones in men whose disease has 'metastased', or spread outside the prostate. The traditional way of doing this was to remove the testicles, which produce most of the testosterone circulating in the bloodstream. The operation, known as orchidectomy (or orchiectomy), is a simple one which can be done under local anaesthetic; but it usually results in impotence and can have a serious psychological effect on the man and his wife.

Sometimes, female hormones (oestrogens such as stilboestrol) are given, which have the effect of suppressing androgen levels, but although not as psychologically traumatizing as castration, oestrogen therapy can cause breast enlargement (gynaecomastia) and fluid retention, and it significantly increases the risk of heart disease and thrombosis.

LHRH agonists and anti-androgens

A more recently developed method of reducing testosterone levels is to use drugs which interfere with the hormonal signal from the brain which stimulates testosterone production in the testes. This hormonal signal is carried by the luteinizing-hormone-releasing hormone (LHRH) originating in the pituitary gland in the brain, which plays a key role in the reproductive process in both men and women. The drugs used, called LHRH agonist analogues, are usually given in the form of subdermal (under the skin) implants, which are renewed every two or three months. Although they do not suppress the androgens produced by the adrenal gland, their use is equivalent to a chemical castration and usually results in impotence. But they are a great improvement on oestrogens, because they do not cause any cardiovascular problems and have less marked feminizing effects. They are however expensive, particularly when compared to orchidectomy, but this should never prevent their use except where cheaper treatment is of equal value to the patient.

One problem in their use is that for the first two or three weeks they cause a sudden surge in androgen levels which results in a 'disease flare'; but thereafter the hormone levels drop quickly to castrate levels.

A promising recent development has been the launch of a 'pure' (non-steroidal) anti-androgen drug, flutamide. This works only at the level of the androgen-dependent secondary sex organs such as the prostate, where it blocks androgen receptors and prevents testosterone-activated growth of prostatic cancer. Flutamide seems to work best in patients with advanced cancer when used in conjunction with an LHRH agonist, or orchidectomy.

Flutamide is usually successful in suppressing the painful 'disease flare' associated with LHRH treatment, and it has little or no effect on libido and sexual potency. Patients taking it feel better, have less pain, fewer urinary problems and a better appetite. Patients with advanced prostatic cancer in a large US study taking flutamide and leuprolide had a longer progression-free survival than patients on LHRH alone; and another study claimed an 88 per cent two-year survival rate for patients with D2 cancer who took the same combination of drugs.

Hyperthermia

The pioneering work done in Israel on the use of hyperthermia in prostate disease, described in Chapter 5, actually started with the treatment of patients with advanced prostate cancer. They found that, in many cases, hyperthermia treatment led to a regression of the tumour and an improvement in voiding: the men were in less pain and had fewer symptoms.

The Israelis' starting point was that hyperthermia (heat a little above blood temperature) has been known for many years to make cancerous cells more susceptible to damage than ordinary cells. This fact has been used to treat surface tumours for some years. If the heated tumours are then subjected to a further assault, from radiotherapy or chemotherapy, they are likely to shrink – possibly even disappear.

It is still too early to say exactly how useful hyperthermia will turn out to be in the treatment of prostatic cancer: its main use may prove to be in the treatment of benign enlargement. But there is considerable interest in its use in conjunction with other therapies such as radiation treatment.

In the United States, the Health Sciences Center at the University of Arizona in Tucson has been experimenting for some years with the use of hyperthermia in combination with external beam and interstitial radiotherapy, with very promising results. Urologists there use hyperthermia generated by ultrasound, rather than microwave, but the effects and the temperature reached (43°C) are similar. They control the temperature very accurately by placing thermocouple probes under local anaesthetic into the prostate tumour through the perineum, guided by transrectal ultrasound.

They are treating patients with C1 and D1 cancers which have not spread outside the pelvis, and some who have had a local recurrence after radical prostatectomy. Heat treatments are given once a week for approximately one and a half hours during the course of external beam radiotherapy. It is early days yet, since the treatment is only experimental, to establish safety and side-effects, and any additional effects of the hyperthermia.

Emotional aspects

Cancer is a frightening word surrounded by fears, myths and silence. As we have seen, 'prostate' has similar connotations. When the two coincide, the effect can be overwhelming. Incontinence, impotence and castration are certainly among the most frightening words to most men – and they are unfortunately all possibilities when prostate cancer is diagnosed.

Different people may go through different feelings in trying to come to terms with their illness. Among common reactions are: shock ('It can't be true'); denial ('There's nothing wrong with me'); anger ('Why me?'); blame and guilt ('It's my own fault'); uncertainty ('Will the treatment work?'); withdrawal ('Please leave me alone'). Wives, friends and family members often need as much support as the man himself.

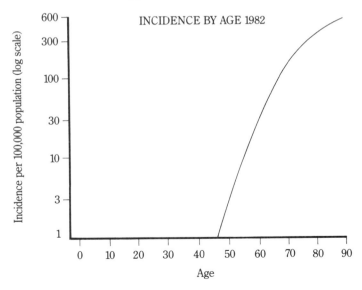

Fig. 8.5: incidence graph of prostate cancer

Prostate disease involves many areas which men of any age find it difficult and embarrassing to talk about and may try to ignore. The first thing to realize, if you are found to have prostate cancer, is that it is best not to bottle things up, but talk about your fears and feelings to your doctors, relatives and friends. The very act of expressing your fears will often make you feel better. Ask your doctor as many questions as you like about your treatment and possible side-effects: your personal problems in connection with your illness are his responsibility too. If you feel unable to cope, there are supporting organizations who can almost certainly help you.

A final thing to remember is that sufferers from cancers and other serious diseases who have a positive approach to their illness usually fare better than patients who languish in depression: 'fighting an illness' has a real meaning and it may well be that a positive outlook helps reinforce the body's natural defence mechanisms and immune responses.

CHAPTER 9

The prostate taboo – prevention and screening – prospects

Men are comparatively lucky in enjoying good health in their sexual and urinary systems, with problems not usually arising until they are relatively old. Prostate problems are rare before the age of 50 and usually do not present problems until men reach their 60s or 70s. Urinary tract infections are comparatively rare, and providing a man does not run the risk of exposing himself to sexually transmitted diseases, so are infections of the sexual organs. Most men remain potent and fertile well into old age, being able to father a child with relative ease in their 60s and even later.

Women fare much worse in all these respects. Women are much more prone to cystitis and recurrent urinary tract infections, mainly because the urethra is much shorter than in men. When a woman has sexual intercourse, especially for the first time, bacteria in the vagina or on the penis can easily be pushed up into the bladder, setting up a painful infection. The length of the male urethra effectively prevents infection unless there is a blockage leading to stale urine accumulating in the bladder, and an antibacterial substance produced by the prostate also helps prevent infections.

When women become infected with a sexually transmitted disease, they also tend to suffer more than men. The symptoms are often less easily recognized, leading to worse infections becoming established before the condition is treated. Such infections can prove stubborn and resistant to treatment, spreading to other sexual organs such as the womb and fallopian tubes and sometimes leading to infertility.

The natural processes of menstruation, pregnancy and

childbirth, while often causing no problems, do lead to complications among many women requiring medical intervention, and women have to be routinely screened and examined throughout pregnancy to guard their health and that of their baby. After childbirth, complications can also arise, as they can at the age of the menopause.

Because of this, most women become used to regular examinations, including internal ones, from a relatively early age and will continue to have check-ups throughout their lives. Most women seek medical advice when they become sexually active in order to use effective contraception, and need regular check-ups if they are using medical methods of birth control. Women will have cervical smear tests, tests during pregnancy, and other medical screening tests throughout their lives. Partly because of all this, and partly because most women are more open in talking to other women about their health, women tend to be more in tune with their bodies and more willing to seek medical advice than men. They tend to view health checks and the doctor–patient relationship rather differently from men, some of whom are proud to boast that they have 'never had to see a doctor in their entire life'.

In the last 20 years or so women have become still more open in discussing matters like antenatal care, menstrual problems, contraceptive methods and their side-effects, gynaecological operations such as hysterectomies and sex-related illnesses such as cystitis and sexually transmitted infections. Articles on these subjects abound in women's magazines, in newspapers and on radio and television health programmes. In contrast, there remains a silence on issues surrounding the male reproductive or urinary systems. Male infertility, prostate problems, and sexual problems such as impotence remain taboo areas which are seldom discussed by men, or by women either. They are talked about in hushed tones, become the subject of jokes, and are viewed by men, women and society in general as somehow distasteful.

One example of this silence concerns male infertility. Because of the confusion in people's minds about the link between virility and fertility, a man who cannot father a child is often seen as impotent or somehow 'less than a man'. Despite the fact that male infertility is just as common as female infertility, there is much less attention focused on it; techniques like *in vitro* fertilization (test tube baby treatment) – which in fact is a boon for male infertility as well as female – seem uniquely debated as the infertile woman's dream-come-true. Artificial insemination by donor is a relatively popular technique, resulting in the birth of around 3,000 babies every year in the UK, but remains surrounded by silence, with very few parents telling the child let alone informing family and friends. Mostly, the wife has to bear the burden, pretending that it is she who is infertile, to save her husband's face.

Even men who have a vasectomy and thus choose to be infertile may find themselves the object of mirth among friends and colleagues, and often have to put the record straight. Many men find all this so difficult and embarrassing that they choose to keep silent about their chosen method of birth control rather than laying themselves open to misunderstandings and jokes.

Similarly, a large number of men feel unable to 'let on' about their prostate problems because they fear this too will reduce their masculinity in the eyes of their friends and lead to jokes behind their backs about being 'past it' now. Unfortunately, because of the ignorance which surrounds the disease and its treatment, such fears are not wholly unfounded. One man who had told his colleagues about his impending prostate surgery, had heard them talking at the coffee machine about what his wife would be getting up to once her old man had 'had the chop'. Others felt that they were treated as objects of pity and even fear, as if the condition were somehow catching.

Unlike women, who form support groups and often remain friends with other sufferers they have met at clinics or in hospital, men tend to remain isolated and alone when it comes to illnesses. They are reluctant on the whole to talk to other men, and they may find their wives are less than sympathetic. Husbands often say that their wives dismiss their fears and accuse them of 'making a fuss' because they, as women, have had to suffer much more pain and discomfort in the course of their lives, especially during pregnancy and childbirth.

It is perhaps time that men 'came out of the closet' a little in dealing with their health problems. Not only would this dispel some of the harmful myths which still circulate, it would enable men to talk more openly and confidently with their doctor or surgeon. By comparing experiences, men could club together and ensure that they get better and more compassionate treatment by doctors in general and urologists in particular.

Preventive measures

As medical attention has increasingly focused on preventing disease rather than simply curing it, the question arises as to whether men, like women, should have regular screening tests or health check-ups to look out for prostate problems, so that they can be treated before they become dangerous. Women have for some years been able to have 'Pap smears' which can identify suspicious cell growth on the cervix and enable treatment to be given before cancer develops. Women can also have mammography scans and are encouraged to carry out breast self-examination for suspicious lumps. The screening system may be criticized, at least in Britain, as being inadequate, but at least it exists.

Some of the risk factors for female cancers are well understood: early promiscuity and exposure to sexually transmitted disease increase the risks of cervical cancer, and relatively early childbearing and full breast-feeding are known to protect against breast cancer. The contraceptive pill, while probably increasing the risk of breast cancer, helps to protect against the rarer but dangerous ovarian cancer.

But the risk factors for prostate disease, whether benign or malignant, are poorly understood. Exposure to sexually transmitted disease and organisms such as chlamydia *may* increase the risk of prostatitis. There has been some suggestion that vasectomy, or exposure to sexually transmitted disease, could increase the risk of developing prostate cancer, but findings are inconclusive. Sexual activity (or the lack of it) seems to have no bearing on the development of prostate disease.

It is known that some racial groups seem less likely to develop benign enlargement or prostate cancer, and the reasons appear to be an interaction of genetic and environmental factors. Some diseases are certainly more common in some ethnic groups, and since male baldness and body hairiness – characteristics which are governed by the same hormone implicated in prostate disease, dihydro-testosterone (DHT) – are to a certain extent genetically predisposed, it would not be surprising to find a genetic link with prostate disease.

As far as benign enlargement is concerned, only some naturopaths claim to be able to prevent or contain the disease through diet and natural remedies. Conventional medicine can so far offer no such hope, although it is possible that the 5-alpha reductase inhibitors described in Chapter 5 may turn out to prevent the development of benign enlargement if taken before the process starts – say, by men in their late 30s. (It could conceivably also stop them going bald as well!)

'Preventive' prostatectomies are occasionally done in some countries, usually on a patient's request, but since no one can be sure that prostate enlargement is going to cause medical problems, this operation is surely no more justified than 'preventive' hysterectomy.

Screening for benign enlargement

Screening for urinary obstruction caused by prostate enlargement is certainly possible, but unlikely to appeal to many men. A rectal examination and flow rate test would reveal most cases, but when surgery is the only treatment, screening is probably not going to be worth while, since few men would choose to undergo surgery 'in case' they developed serious symptoms.

'Do-it-yourself' screening requires honesty and common sense but could undoubtedly perform a useful function. Flow-rate assessment can be done quite satisfactorily at home. Disposal urine flow meters can be ordered quite cheaply from the chemist's: essentially they are graduated plastic bags with a syphon device for measuring 'peak flow'. It is important that the bladder is full (but not overstretched) in order for a correct reading to be obtained. If the volume of urine passed is under 150 ml, the peak flow reading will not be accurate. No straining should be employed during the test – it will not in any case improve the flow rate. If the flow rate is under 15 ml per second, it is likely that some obstruction is present. The procedure for home rectal examination is described below under 'Cancer screening'.

When there are established non-surgical treatments which can prevent the condition from becoming so serious that surgery is inevitable, screening for benign enlargement would become a far more attractive proposition; this development is certainly a real possibility within the next 10 years.

For the time being, public information and freer discussion

of the condition would probably be the most useful approach, with the objective of preventing the tragedies occurring when men put off seeking medical advice about their prostate problems early enough and suffer kidney damage as a result.

However, screening for prostate cancer is a distinct possibility. The disease is one of the cancers causing the most fatalities among men, and although most men dying of the disease are elderly, prevention of the advance of prostate cancer through screening and detection in its early stages is clearly attractive.

Screening for prostate cancer

Urologists are divided on the need for widespread screening for cancer of the prostate. As was mentioned above, large numbers of men have prostate cancer without knowing it, and most go to their graves without being troubled by it. Yet if early cancer was detected in younger men – who may have a life expectancy of 25 years – there is good reason to think that mortality from this disease could be reduced. At present it accounts for some 7,000 deaths a year in the UK – around 2.2 per cent of all male deaths. However, only some 600 deaths a year occur in men under 65.

Of the over 8,000 new cases diagnosed in the UK every year, only just over a third are alive five years later. The reason for this is largely late diagnosis – in up to 70 per cent of all newly diagnosed cases, the disease has already spread outside the gland and is consequently, in most cases, incurable.

Another consideration is that any treatment given must not be worse for the patient than the disease itself. Methods of identifying patients with cancer must be found so that innocuous tumours can merely be closely observed for changes, while the more dangerous tumours can be treated aggressively. No one yet knows if early detection and treatment can have a significant effect on the alarming death rate – but it seems likely.

In many countries, men over 40 are routinely given a rectal examination. In the United States, it is always included in a medical examination and is compulsory for men in the armed services, and in West Germany and Austria it is available free to all men over 45. France and Italy have recently started a similar scheme. In Germany, under a quarter of men participated in the programme, and only around 2 per cent have suspicious findings. Since the proportion of positive biopsies in suspicious prostates is only about 15 per cent, the number of cancers revealed must be small.

However, in the United States the number of prostate cancer deaths expressed as a proportion of new prostate cancer cases is far smaller than in Britain. A 1990 report of the British Office of Population Censuses and Surveys comparing the chances of surviving cancer in the United Kingdom and the United States showed that only 36 per cent of men with prostate cancer survived beyond five years in England and Wales, compared with 65 per cent of American men with diagnosed prostate cancer. This can only mean that more early cases are detected, and cured, in that country.

The rectal examination is not foolproof – the doctor's finger can only detect tumours over a certain size, on the part of the gland that he can reach. But this is how most prostate cancers are still diagnosed, and the examination, while slightly distasteful, is really not painful and is over very quickly.

A more accurate method of screening is by using transrectal ultrasound (see Chapter 1). Instead of the doctor's finger, an ultrasound probe is placed in the rectum and the images examined on the screen. It can detect tumours as small as 5mm in diameter (under a quarter of an inch). Any suspected abnormality can then be accurately confirmed by ultrasound-guided biopsy. But the equipment is expensive and it is difficult to operate. At present only a few centres have it or the staff capable of operating it. What is more, it is difficult to distinguish on the ultrasound scan between certain types of prostatitis and cancer, so there are many false positives.

Another type of scan which can theoretically show abnormalities likely to be missed in a rectal examination is computed tomography (CT) scanning. But the equipment for this is even more expensive, and moreover seems to be less effective than transrectal ultrasound. Magnetic Resonance Imaging (MRI) is expensive too, and at present offers little advantage, but there are hopes that further refinements of this type of scan could improve its usefulness in the future.

A blood test to measure the level of an enzyme called the prostate-specific antigen (PSA) can be done, but this is mainly useful in detecting whether cancer has spread outside the prostate itself – so not much help in detecting early disease.

It has been suggested that men could be taught how to do rectal self-examination: one well-known surgeon used to perform it on himself regularly. It seems unlikely that many men would be prepared to do this, but a more reasonable alternative is examination by a friend or family member.

For this the man kneels on the floor with his chest and abdomen over a bed. The examiner should wear a surgical glove and lubricate the forefinger with a sterile gel such as Vaseline. He or she should press the examining finger against the man's anus, wait for the external muscles to relax, then gently but firmly insert the finger to its limit and press downwards lightly with the pad of the finger to feel the prostate. The prostate should feel smooth and firm and the examiner should be able to detect the midline groove (sulcus). The muscle between the base of the thumb and forefinger of a clenched fist gives an idea of the normal consistency of the prostate. If the prostate feels lumpy and very hard, then medical advice should be sought.

Health-screening generally is more common in North America than in Britain, where it tends to be limited to workplace screening, mainly of directors and management. More facilities are available for women, no doubt for the reasons outlined earlier in this chapter. Perhaps there is a case for setting up some pilot 'Well Man' clinics, which could screen for cardiovascular and lung diseases common in men as well as prostate disease. Prostate screening could also include routine examination of the genitalia to screen for testicular tumours and varicocele (a usually curable cause of male infertility), and a urine test to detect renal and bladder cancer.

While men, rightly or wrongly, would not be strongly motivated to volunteer for such screening as long as surgery is virtually the only treatment available for prostate enlargement, it would be a different story if the screening was likely to result in treatment which would *avoid* surgery.

It seems likely that within a very few years this will be the case. The hyperthermia therapy, pills and stents described in Chapter 5 are likely to be more widely available within a matter of years. Urologists, though generally conservative and surgeons by training and thinking, will have to adapt to non-surgical methods, or lose their patients. Preventive and minimally invasive medicine is in the ascendant, and economics and the increasing need to reduce the demand for hospital beds will force even the British National Health Service – hidebound in a different way from the medical profession itself – to give more serious attention to preventive screening and innovative outpatient therapies.

The patient himself can hasten this process by nudging and badgering his doctor, consultant and hospital, because the conservatism of the profession is deeply ingrained. In 1909, when a revolutionary new device, the Brown Buerger cystoscope (for visual examination of the inside of the bladder), was first described by Hurry Fenwick at the Medical Society of London, the audience of distinguished surgeons laughed out loud. Every sensible surgeon knew perfectly well that the only way to examine the bladder was to cut into the urethra and pass a finger through it to feel the inside of the bladder: cystoscopy was obviously rubbish. Transurethral prostatectomy was similarly dismissed by most British urologists when it was first introduced from the United States.

The promising treatments now being developed – hyperthermia and DHT-inhibitors – have also been sceptically received. But there are always more progressive consultants who have open minds and a less blinkered view of where the interests of their patients really lie, and they in time will win over the majority of their profession to the really worthwhile innovations.

It is important not to make one's doctor or consultant feel that they are being outflanked by a 'know-all' patient: there is nothing they hate worse. But a well-informed patient does not have to be threatening, and a good doctor will always be prepared to inform himself about a drug or a treatment he is unfamiliar with. Patients should not forget that most doctors and consultants work long hours and, unless they are at teaching hospitals, cannot be expected to have read of all the latest medical developments.

To sum up, medical treatment for the most common male complaint of benign enlargement, and to a lesser extent for prostate cancer and prostatitis too, is at a turning point, and it will pay all men – and their doctors – to know what treatments are likely to be available in the next few years and what their consequences are likely to be for men's reproductive and general health.

Further reading

There are practically no other non-technical books on prostate problems in the English language in print. The only thorough book for the general reader, which contains more medical detail on some topics than the present book, is one by an American urologist:

The Prostate Book: Sound advice on symptoms and treatment Stephen Rous MD (W. W. Norton, New York and London, 1989).

The most recent academic book on the subject (although already out of date in certain respects) is:

The Prostate, edited by John M. Fitzpatrick and Robert J. Krane (Churchill Livingstone, Edinburgh, London, Melbourne and New York, 1989).

Readers interested in pursuing naturopathic remedies and diets (although some of the book's medical statements and claims should be viewed with a critical eye) may like to consult:

Prostate Troubles Leon Chaitow ND, DO (Thorsons (New Self-Help Series), 1988).

An excellent book on the general subject of male sexual health is:

Men's Reproductive Health, edited by Janice M. Swanson and Katherine A. Forrest (Springer Publishing, New York, 1984).

A useful free booklet on prostate cancer is:

Understanding Cancer of the Prostate, British Association of Cancer United Patients (BACUP), 121/123 Charterhouse Street, London EC1M 6AA (1987).

A good general book on cancer and the emotional problems it brings is:

Cancer: Your Life, Your Choice Rachael Clyne (Thorsons, 1986).

Index